Endocrinopathy after Childhood Cancer Treatment

Endocrine Development

Vol. 15

Series Editor

P.-E. Mullis Bern

Endocrinopathy after Childhood Cancer Treatment

Volume Editors

W.H.B. Wallace Edinburgh
C.J.H. Kelnar Edinburgh

21figures, 4 in color, and 11 tables, 2009

KARGER

Basel · Freiburg · Paris · London · New York · Bangalore · Bangkok · Shanghai · Singapore · Tokyo · Sydney

Endocrine Development

Founded 1999 by Martin O. Savage, London

Dr. W. Hamish B. Wallace, MD, FRCP, FRCPCH
Department of Paediatric Oncology
Section of Child Life and Health
Royal Hospital for Sick Children
University of Edinburgh
Edinburgh, UK

Prof. Christopher J.H. Kelnar, MA, MD, FRCP, FRCPCH
Department of Paediatric Endocrinology
Section of Child Life and Health
Royal Hospital for Sick Children
University of Edinburgh
Edinburgh, UK

Library of Congress Cataloging-in-Publication Data

Endocrinopathy after childhood cancer treatment / volume editors, W.H.B. Wallace, C.J.H. Kelnar.
p. ; cm. – (Endocrine development, ISSN 1421-7082; v. 15)
Includes bibliographical references and indexes.
ISBN 978-3-8055-9037-2 (hard cover: alk. Paper)
1. Cancer in children–Treatment–Complications. 2. Cancer in children–Treatment–Endocrine aspects.
I. Wallace, Hamish. II. Kelnar, C.J.H. III. Series: Endocrine development; v. 15.
[DNLM: 1. Endocrine System Diseases–etiology. 2. Neoplasms–therapy. 3. Antineoplastic Agents–adverse effects. 4. Bone Marrow Transplantation–adverse effects. 5. Child. 6. Radiotherapy–adverse effects. 7. Surgical Procedures, Operative–adverse effects.
W1 EN3635 v.15 2009 / WS 330 E568 2009]
RC281.C4E53 2009
618.92'994–dc22

2008052186

Bibliographic Indices. This publication is listed in bibliographic services, including Current Contents® and PubMed/MEDLINE.

www.karger.com
Printed in Switzerland on acid-free and non-aging paper (ISO 9706) by Reinhardt Druck, Basel
ISSN 1421–7082
ISBN 978–3–8055–9037–2
e-ISBN 978–3–8055–9038–9

Contents

Foreword

This volume brings together two editors, Dr. Hamish Wallace, an oncologist, and Prof. Christopher Kelnar, an endocrinologist, who work closely together at the Royal Hospital for Sick Children in Edinburgh, UK. They have assembled an impressive list of international contributors to discuss experiences and review the latest scientific advances on key clinical topics related to childhood cancer therapy. As written in the Preface, this is a field which is constantly evolving and this volume offers a very relevant update. The editors have carefully put the care of the patient first and the chapters, which cover all the important areas of late-effects endocrinopathy, examine the evidence-base which is now available to optimize long-term care of childhood cancer survivors.

I am delighted to welcome this volume to the *Endocrine Development* series. It makes an excellent contribution to the series which it has been my privilege to edit during the last 7 years.

Martin O. Savage, London

Preface

Continuing advances in the management of childhood malignancies mean that the majority of children treated for cancer can realistically expect long-term survival and, indeed, nearly 1 in 700 of the adult population are now childhood cancer survivors. However, children, young people and adult survivors experience morbidity which is generally related to the treatment they received to cure their cancer (surgery, neurosurgery, radiotherapy, chemotherapy and/or bone marrow transplantation) rather than to the cancer itself. The challenges for doctors and other healthcare professionals looking after these patients is to sustain and further increase survival rates whilst reducing the incidence and severity of such treatment-induced 'late effects'.

Morbidities in this group of patients include second cancers, neurodevelopmental, cognitive and psychological problems, and renal, respiratory and hepatic dysfunction, but much significant but anticipatable, preventable and/or treatable morbidity is in the areas of growth impairment, puberty progression, fertility and diverse endocrine dysfunction. The prevention, diagnosis and management of growth-, puberty- and endocrine-related morbidity is thus of major and increasing importance.

There is an increasing, and increasingly rigorous, evidence-base behind the diagnosis and management of these problems but still much controversy over pathophysiology, optimal investigative and management protocols and follow-up strategies. In this volume leaders in the field of childhood cancer late effects bring a variety of clinical perspectives to the examination of these issues with chapters re-evaluating the effects of childhood cancer therapies on growth, puberty and hypothalamic and pituitary function, male and female fertility, obesity, and metabolic and bone problems, and discussion of long-term follow-up issues and strategies.

We thank our fellow contributors and hope that this volume will be of particular interest to paediatric endocrinologists, adult and reproductive endocrinologists, primary care practitioners, nurses and nurse practitioners and others involved in the planning and delivery of the holistic care which this increasingly numerous and important group of patients require.

W. Hamish B. Wallace, Edinburgh
Christopher J.H. Kelnar, Edinburgh

Wallace WHB, Kelnar CJH (eds): Endocrinopathy after Childhood Cancer Treatment.
Endocr Dev. Basel, Karger, 2009, vol 15, pp 1–24

Hypopituitarism following Radiotherapy Revisited

Ken H. Darzy · Stephen M. Shalet

Department of Endocrinology, Christie Hospital NHS Trust, Manchester, UK

Abstract

Neuroendocrine disturbances in anterior pituitary hormone secretion are common following radiation damage to the hypothalamic-pituitary (H-P) axis, the severity and frequency of which correlate with the total radiation dose delivered to the H-P axis and the length of follow-up. The somatotropic axis is the most vulnerable to radiation damage and GH deficiency remains the most frequently seen endocrinopathy. Compensatory hyperstimulation of a partially damaged somatotropic axis may restore normality of spontaneous GH secretion in the context of reduced but normal stimulated responses in adults. At its extreme, endogenous hyperstimulation may limit further stimulation by insulin-induced hypoglycaemia resulting in subnormal GH responses despite the normality of spontaneous GH secretion. In children, failure of the hyperstimulated partially damaged H-P axis to meet the increased demands for GH during growth and puberty may explain what has previously been described as radiation-induced GH neurosecretory dysfunction and, unlike in adults, the insulin tolerance test remains the gold standard for assessing H-P functional reserve. With low radiation doses (<30 Gy) GH deficiency usually occurs in isolation in about 30% of patients, while with radiation doses of 30–50 Gy, the incidence of GH deficiency can reach 50–100% and long-term gonadotropin, TSH and ACTH deficiencies occur in 20–30, 3–9 and 3–6% of patients, respectively. With higher dose cranial irradiation (>60 Gy) or following conventional irradiation for pituitary tumours (30–50 Gy), multiple hormonal deficiencies occur in 30–60% after 10 years of follow-up. Precocious puberty can occur after radiation doses of <30 Gy in girls only, and in both sexes equally with a radiation dose of 30–50 Gy. Hyperprolactinaemia, due to hypothalamic damage is mostly seen in young women after high dose cranial irradiation and is usually subclinical. H-P dysfunction is progressive and irreversible and can have an adverse impact on growth, body image, sexual function and quality of life. Regular testing is advised to ensure timely diagnosis and early hormone replacement therapy.

Neuroendocrine abnormalities may follow external cranial radiotherapy given for a variety of brain tumours and haematological malignancies when the hypothalamic-pituitary (H-P) axis lies within the radiation field. Radiation-induced anterior pituitary hormone deficiencies are the most common long-term complications of successful cancer treatment. They are irreversible and progressive and negatively impact on growth, skeletal health, sexual function and fertility, and ultimately, quality of life. Regular testing is, thus, important to achieve timely diagnosis and to aid the introduction of appropriate hormone replacement therapy to prevent or ameliorate these adverse consequences.

Radiobiology

The neurotoxicity of any radiation schedule is a function of the total radiation dose, the fraction size and the time allowed between fractions for tissue repair (duration of the radiation schedule). To minimise the damage to healthy neuronal tissues (including the H-P axis), most radiation schedules have not used more than 2 Gy per fraction and no more than 5 fractions per week. Increasing the fraction size above 2 Gy per fraction (for the same total dose) can induce relatively more injury to the late responding (neuronal) than the early responding (tumour) tissues [1]. Thus, a typical cranial irradiation schedule of 30–50 Gy administered to a pituitary or non-pituitary brain tumour will take 3–5 weeks to complete. Similarly, total body irradiation (TBI) with a dose of 10–16 Gy is typically given in 3–8 fractions. Neurotoxicity also depends on the nature of the tissue/cells irradiated and their vulnerability to radiation damage. This is clearly accounted for in the calculation of the biological effective dose, which is a standardised means to compare the intensity and biological impact of various radiation schedules [1] and to predict the development of anterior pituitary hormone deficiencies, particularly GH deficiency (GHD) [2–4].

Pathophysiology and Site of Radiation Damage

The pathophysiology of radiation-induced damage remains poorly understood and most conclusions have been based on clinical observations in man, with only a few studies in animal models. Chieng et al. [5] concluded that direct injury to the H-P cells, rather than reduced hypothalamic blood flow, is the major cause of progressive h-P dysfunction after fractionated cranial irradiation. They showed that regional hypothalamic blood flow after cranial irradiation was reduced. However, there was no significant difference in the hypothalamic/occipital blood flow ratio between 6 months and 5 years after irradiation, in stark contrast to the progressive endocrine dysfunction with time in these patients. Further objective evidence for direct neuronal damage came from the observations of Hochberg et al. [6]

who studied rat pituitary cell survival and GH secretion after in vitro irradiation of pituitary cell cultures. Their data reveal the marked sensitivity of the somatotropes to single doses of radiation as low as 300 cGy and the remarkable resistance of the gonadotropin- and TSH-secreting cells to doses as high as 1,000 cGy. Evidence for direct neuronal damage is also provided by the remarkable difference in the incidence of anterior pituitary hormone deficiencies, which is consistent with direct radiation-induced selective hypothalamic neuronal and pituitary cell damage rather than a universal insult to the H-P axis. Thus, differential radiosensitivity of H-P function has been proposed and clinical observations reveal that the GH axis is the most radiosensitive followed by the gonadotropin, ACTH and TSH axes. These observations in humans are similar to those seen in experimental animal models by Hochberg et al. [6] and more recently by Robinson et al. [7]. In the latter study, differential radiosensitivity of H-P function and the dose and time dependency of anterior pituitary hormone deficiencies were clearly demonstrated in young adult rats. In this experiment, changes in pituitary hormone contents were analysed. GH and PRL were most sensitive and decreased by more than 90% after irradiation. TSH contents were unaffected 8 weeks after the lowest dose of irradiation, but were reduced at 14 and 20 weeks. LH and ACTH were the slowest to be affected, and then only at the higher doses of radiation.

Thus, variable degrees of GHD are usually seen in isolation after lower radiation doses used in patients with leukaemia or brain tumours (18–50 Gy) [8–12]. However, with more intensive irradiation schedules used in particular for the treatment of nasopharyngeal carcinoma (NPC) and skull base tumours (>60 Gy), other (relatively more radioresistant) neuroendocrine axes are affected leading to early and multiple pituitary hormone deficits [11, 13–15]. In patients with NPC but no skull base invasion, it has been shown that modification of the radiotherapy technique to provide shielding of the H-P axis from the irradiated target volume resulted in no neuroendocrine complications after a median follow-up of 31.5 months compared with an 11% complication rate in the unshielded group without jeopardising local control [16].

The conclusions regarding how age influences the impact of radiation on H-P function are conflicting. Early observations of independent studies reporting the frequency of GHD following well-defined radiation schedules suggested that younger age increases vulnerability to radiation damage. In this context, GHD, as defined by a subnormal response to the insulin tolerance test (ITT), was seen frequently in children treated with TBI [17] but in none of the adults who had received comparable TBI schedules [18]. In addition, it was suggested that younger children receiving prophylactic cranial irradiation for acute lymphoblastic leukaemia are more susceptible to radiation-induced GHD than older children [19]. Similarly, in their study of 166 patients aged 6–80 years who had received high dose irradiation for tumours of the head and neck, Samaan et al. [20] showed that children younger than 15 years of age had a higher incidence of GHD soon after radiotherapy than older patients; however, the older age group showed more ACTH and LH deficiency. These observations have been reinforced by Agha et al. [4] who reported variable degrees of hypopituitarism in 41% of 56 patients irradiated for non-pituitary brain tumours in adulthood. In this study [4], GHD (32%) was less frequent than that reported in irradiated children [9, 20, 21], but ACTH (21%), TSH (9%) and gonadotropin (27%) deficiencies were relatively more common or similar in frequency to that reported in cancer survivors irradiated during childhood [3, 8, 20, 21]. Thus, it appears that age may influence the various H-P axis susceptibility to radiation damage differentially.

The predominant site of radiation damage, pituitary vs. hypothalamic, has attracted some controversy. In the higher range of conventional irradiation, i.e. doses of >60 Gy, there is robust clinical evidence to suggest that radiation inflicts dual damage to both the pituitary as well as the hypothalamus resulting in early multiple anterior pituitary hormone deficiencies. Pituitary damage is demonstrated by impaired GH, LH/FSH, and TSH responses to direct stimulation with exogenous GHRH, LHRH or TRH, respectively. Hypothalamic damage, on the other hand, is characterised by a hypothalamic pattern of responses (delayed responses) to LHRH and TRH tests and more importantly, the occurrence of hyperprolactinaemia due to a reduction in hypothalamic release of the inhibitory neurotransmitter, dopamine. These abnormalities have been clearly described in those intensively irradiated for NPC [11, 15, 22] and skull base tumours [13, 20] but much less frequently in those treated for other brain tumours or leukaemia with less intensive radiation schedules [8, 23]. With radiation doses of <40 Gy and particularly following prophylactic cranial irradiation for leukaemia (18–24 Gy), where GHD is usually the only manifestation of radiation damage, it has been previously suggested that the hypothalamus might be the predominant site of radiation damage with time-dependent somatotrope dysfunction occurring as a result of secondary somatotrope atrophy due to reduced hypothalamic GHRH release. This belief was based on the results of many studies that showed relative preservation of GH responses to direct stimulation of the pituitary with exogenous GHRH in the context of impaired responses to insulin-induced hypoglycaemia. However, recent studies by the authors of stimulated and spontaneous GH secretion in adult cancer survivors, which are detailed in the next section, have strongly suggested the opposite with robust evidence that direct radiation-induced damage to the pituitary still occurs even with low radiation doses and that the pituitary may be the predominant site of radiation damage [24]. These conclusions are in accord with earlier observations that showed marked sensitivity of the somatotropes after in vitro irradiation of rat pituitary cell culture with single doses as low as 300 cGy [6] and more recently the in vitro studies, which showed that radiation doses of 20–50 Gy were capable of inducing apoptosis of rat pituitary cell lines [25].

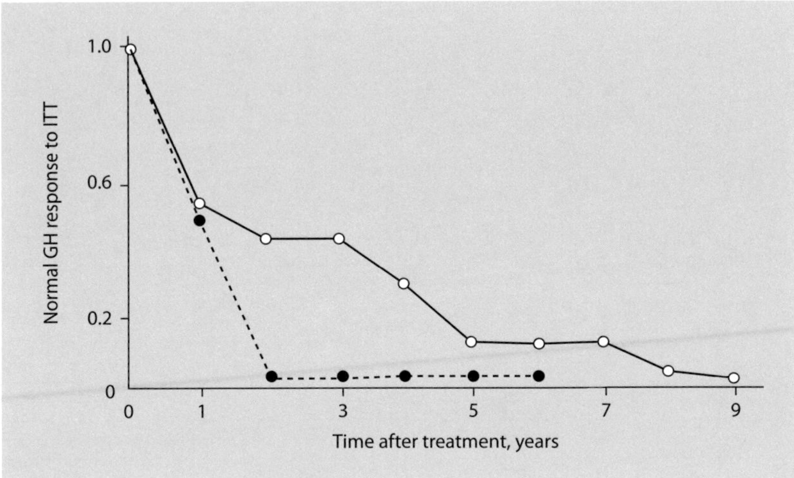

Fig. 1. The incidence of GH deficiency in children receiving 27–32 Gy (○—○) or ≥35 Gy (●- - -●) cranial irradiation for a brain tumour in relation to time from irradiation. Reproduced with permission from Clayton and Shalet [9].

H-P dysfunction secondary to radiation is also time dependent with both the increased incidence and severity of hormonal deficits with longer post-irradiation follow-up intervals [3, 9, 26, 27]. The progressive nature of the hormonal deficits following radiation damage to the H-P axis (fig. 1, 2) can be attributed to secondary pituitary atrophy consequent upon lack of hypothalamic releasing/tropic factors, especially after intensive irradiation that undoubtedly inflicts hypothalamic damage, and/or delayed direct effects of radiotherapy on the axis. The latter is supported by the gradual decline in the elevated prolactin levels seen in some patients after prolonged periods of follow-up [28]. In addition to pituitary cell death induced by radiation [25], the latter also causes diffuse fibrosis in the adenohypophysis, but not the neurohypophysis, with an increased number of folliculostellate cells. This may contribute to the progressive neuroendocrine dysfunction, in addition to any contribution from radiation-induced mitochondrial dysfunction and squamous metaplasia in the actual pituitary endocrine cells [29].

Hypothalamic damage may not necessarily result in reduced release of tropic factors but may compromise hypothalamic reserve and reduced capacity to respond optimally to the reduced pituitary reserve induced by direct radiation damage. In this context, conventional irradiation schedules with doses that are known to cause mostly isolated GHD in patients with non-pituitary brain tumours, can substantially increase the incidence and severity of anterior pituitary hormone deficiencies when the H-P neuronal integrity/reserve is compromised by a tumour and/or previous surgery [28, 30]. Thus the reported prevalence of pituitary hormone

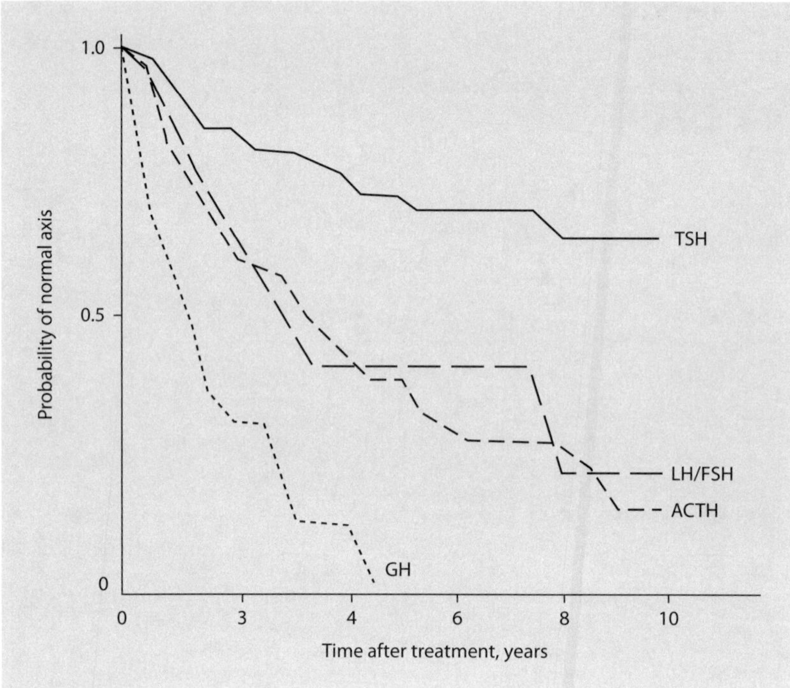

Fig. 2. Life-table analysis indicating probabilities of initially normal hypothalamic-pituitary-target gland axes remaining normal after radiotherapy. Adapted with permission from Littley et al. [28].

deficits following conventional irradiation (30–50 Gy) in patients with pituitary tumours and/or following pituitary surgery [28, 30] are equivalent to the effects of intensive radiation schedules (50–70 Gy) in patients with non-pituitary brain tumours [11, 14, 15] (fig. 2, table 1).

Abnormalities of GH Secretion and GHD

The somatotropic axis is the most vulnerable to radiation damage and GHD is usually the first and is frequently the only manifestation of neuroendocrine injury following cranial irradiation. The severity and speed of onset of radiation-induced GHD is dose-dependent and the incidence increases with time elapsed post-irradiation; nearly 100% of children treated with radiation doses of >30 Gy will have blunted GH responses to the ITT, whilst 35% of those receiving <30 Gy still show a normal peak GH response to the ITT between 2 and 5 years after radiotherapy [9] (fig. 1). Isolated GHD is seen after low dose (18–24 Gy) cranial irradiation [31, 32] more frequently in children than in adults [19] and after TBI with doses

Table 1. Summary of neuroendocrine dysfunction following radiotherapy

Condition treated	Radiation schedule	Neuroendocrine dysfunction and deficiencies
Leukaemia and lymphoma	Fractionated TBI (7–16 Gy)	Isolated GHD, mostly in pubertal children
Leukaemia and lymphoma	Fractionated prophylactic cranial irradiation (18–24 Gy)	(1) Isolated GHD (<30% of children only) (2) Pubertal GH insufficiency (3) Compensated GHD in adults[1] (4) Increased spontaneous cortisol secretion[2] (5) Precocious puberty (in girls only)
Non-pituitary brain tumours	Conventional fractionated cranial irradiation (30–50 Gy)	(1) GHD (30–100%) (2) Compensated GHD in adults[1] (3) Precocious puberty (in both sexes) (4) Gonadotropin deficiency in >20% (long-term) (5) TSH deficiency (3–9% long-term) (6) Subtle abnormalities in TSH secretion (30%) (7) ACTH deficiency (3% long-term) (8) Increased spontaneous cortisol secretion[2] (9) Hyperprolactinaemia (5–20% mostly in women)[3]
Naso-pharyngeal carcinoma and skull base tumours	Conventional fractionated cranial irradiation (50–70 Gy)	(1) GHD (almost in all patients after 5 years) (2) Gonadotropin deficiency (20–50% long-term) (3) TSH deficiency (up to 60% long-term) (4) ACTH deficiency (27–35% long-term) (5) Hyperprolactinaemia (20–50%, mostly in women)[3]
Pituitary tumours	Conventional fractionated cranial irradiation (30–50 Gy)	(1) GHD (almost in all patients after 5 years) (2) Gonadotropin deficiency (up to 60% after 10 years) (3) TSH deficiency (up to 30% after 10 years) (4) ACTH deficiency (up to 60% after 10 years) (5) Hyperprolactinemia (20–50%, mostly in women)[3]

[1] Compensated GHD refers to subnormal stimulated but normal spontaneous GH secretion.
[2] Increased spontaneous cortisol secretion and levels in the context of normal responses to ITT.
[3] Hyperprolactinaemia is often subclinical and rarely seen in children; it diminishes and can normalise with time due to slowly evolving radiation-induced damage of the lactotropes.

as low as 10 Gy in children only [17, 32–34]. Thus, the somatotropic axis is more radiosensitive in children and even with higher radiation doses GHD appears to be much less frequent (around 30%) if irradiation is administered during adulthood [4].

Prospective studies also suggest that impaired GH responses to provocative tests can occur as early as 1 month after high dose radiation therapy (>60 Gy) for

NPC [15] and after 3 months and certainly in the first 12 months after irradiation for brain tumours [12, 35].

In contrast to previous findings in children reported by Clayton and Shalet [9], recent studies have revealed that more than 20% of an unselected cohort of adult survivors of childhood brain tumours had normal GH status more than 10 years after radiotherapy [3, 36]. This apparent discrepancy is not related to recovery of GH status, but can be attributed in part to the use of more strict thresholds for the diagnosis of GHD in adults.

It is generally agreed that the diagnosis of isolated GHD can only be robustly achieved if patients fail to pass at least two GH provocative tests that preferably induce GH release through different mechanisms [37]. Radiation-induced H-P axis dysfunction represents a pathology in which discordant GH responses to mechanistically different provocative tests may be observed raising the question of which test reflects the true GH status. It has been suggested that radiation with doses of <40 Gy causes predominant hypothalamic damage with GHRH deficiency. This hypothesis is based on relative preservation or 'normality' of responses to direct pituitary stimulation with exogenous GHRH compared with other provocative tests, especially the ITT [26, 27, 38–41]. The ITT has therefore been considered the 'gold standard' and frequently stated to be a more robust and sensitive test to identify radiation-induced GHD [42], such that a failed response to the ITT in cranially irradiated patients may be accepted as diagnostic of GHD without resort to further testing. However, this assumption was never objectively confirmed by demonstrating impaired spontaneous GH secretion in those who showed discordant responses [26, 27, 38–41]. Other studies showed discordantly normal or less severely attenuated peak GH responses to arginine stimulation test (AST) compared with the responses to the ITT [42–46], a combination even more difficult to explain by a simple model assuming GHRH deficiency after radiotherapy. Similarly, the combined GHRH+AST also generated discordantly higher GH responses compared with the ITT with a progressive decline in responses with a longer post-irradiation interval [3].

Subsequently, this simplistic hypothesis that radiation-induced GHD is primarily related to hypothalamic damage and GHRH deficiency was contradicted by the finding that radiation mostly inflicted quantitative damage to the H-P axis with preserved GH pulsatility and diurnal variation, albeit with profound amplitude reduction in those in whom the diagnosis of GHD was confirmed unequivocally by virtue of failing severely both the ITT and the GHRH+AST [47] (fig. 3). As GHRH is essential for pulse generation as well as nocturnal augmentation in GH release [48, 49] and pulsatility [50], these findings cast doubt upon the initial theory that the hypothalamus is more radiosensitive, and that radiation (<40 Gy) causes predominantly hypothalamic damage with GHRH deficiency of adequate severity to result in secondary somatotrope atrophy. This assumption was further

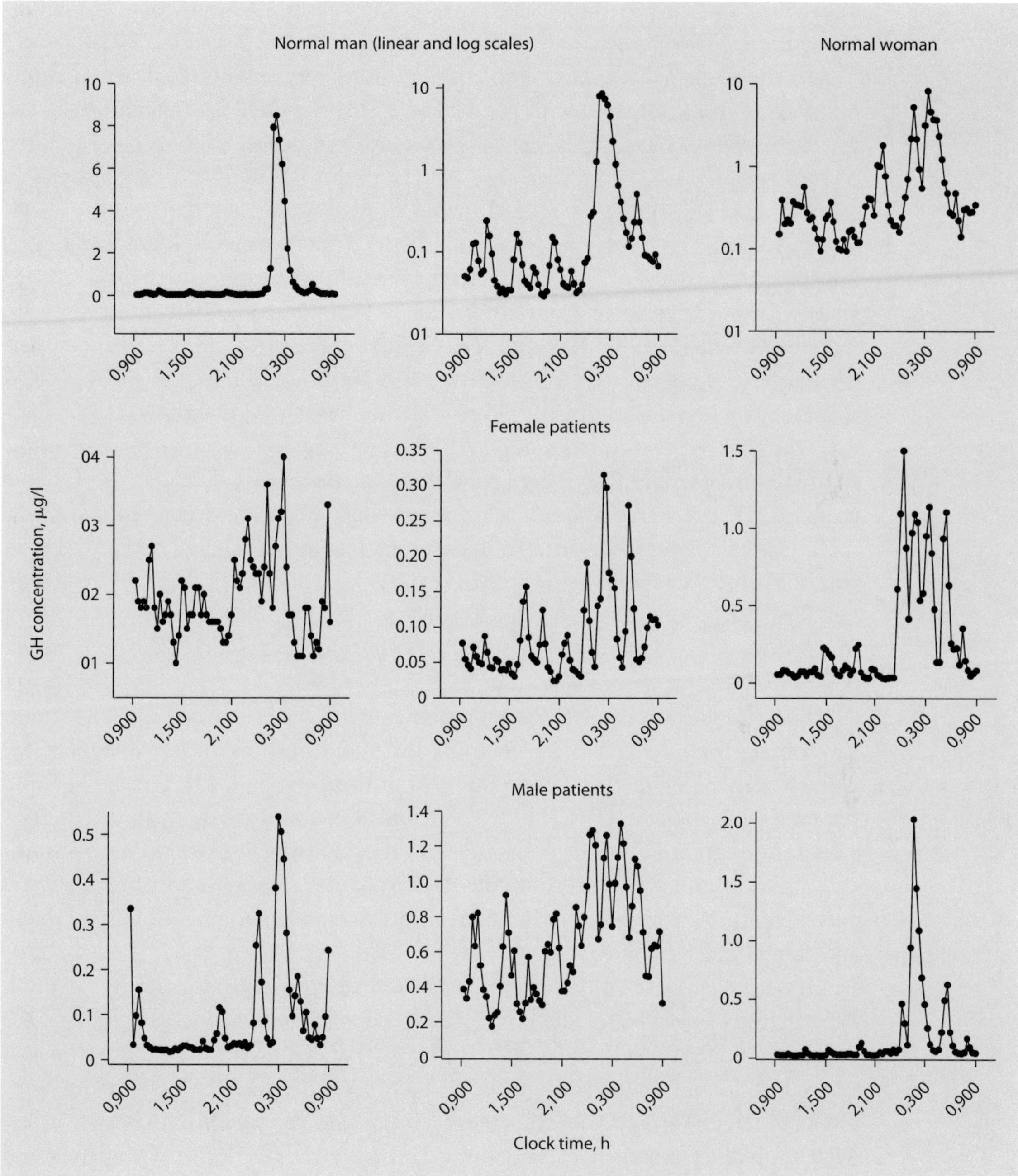

Fig. 3. GH profiles from 2 normal individuals and 6 patients with severe radiation-induced GH deficiency showing the preservation of GH pulsatility and diurnal variation in the patients despite extreme peak amplitude attenuation. Note that most peaks in the patients and many in the normals are below the detection limit of conventional GH assays (0.5 µg/l). Note the relatively higher inter-peak and day GH levels in the women and some patients leading to amplitude dampening of the diurnal variation. Reproduced with permission from Darzy et al. [47].

undermined when physiological GH secretion was studied in a cohort of irradiated patients in whom the individual responses to the ITT and the GHRH+AST were entirely normal but the overall group responses were found to be significantly reduced by 50% compared with gender- and BMI-matched normal controls [24], yet the individual and overall spontaneous GH secretion was fully maintained both in the fed and fasting state (fig. 4). The preservation of spontaneous GH in the context of substantially reduced somatotrope reserve argues against the observations being solely explained by hypothalamic damage with GHRH deficiency, as the combined effects of reduced GHRH secretion with consequent somatotrope atrophy would be expected to result in reduced spontaneous GH secretion. It was, therefore, concluded that radiation causes dual damage to both the pituitary and the hypothalamus and that normality of GH secretion is maintained by a compensatory increase in stimulatory hypothalamic input, i.e. increased GHRH secretion from the residual functioning GHRH-secreting neurons with overdrive of the residual somatotropes [24]. These conclusions are in accord with the experimental models of in vitro irradiation of rat pituitary cells [6, 25], as described above and the infrequent/rare occurrence of hyperprolactinaemia (characteristic marker of hypothalamic damage), after low dose (<40 Gy) irradiation as opposed to its high frequency after intensive (>40 Gy) irradiation [11, 14, 51]. Reduction in somatotrope mass is evident morphologically with significant decreases in pituitary height and volume demonstrated by MRI studies [52].

Thus, the previous belief that radiation causes GHRH deficiency and secondary somatotrope deficiency has become untenable and imprecise to explain the pattern of discordant stimulated responses in some patients who fail the ITT and pass the GHRH or the GHRH+AST. The extent of radiation damage at these two sites and the intensity of the compensatory mechanisms must vary between individuals and ultimately determine the pattern of GH responses to various stimuli and the nature of discordance between stimulated and spontaneous GH secretion at different phases of life.

These novel observations beg the question of how, mechanistically, radiation damage causes relatively better preserved GH responses to GHRH, AST or the combined GHRH+AST rather than to the ITT, and for clinical practice, the precise GH status in those who fail the ITT but pass the GHRH, AST or the combined GHRH+AST. To this end, the findings of a recent study [53] shed some light; individual and overall spontaneous GH secretions were entirely normal both in the fed and fasting state in 5 of 7 patients who had normal GH responses to the GHRH+AST but subnormal responses to the ITT. These findings imply that severely impaired GH responses to the ITT in the context of normal or mildly impaired responses to the GHRH+AST may reflect the presence of endogenous hyperactivation of the H-P axis resulting in partial or complete restoration of spontaneous GH secretion, depending on the residual mass of functioning

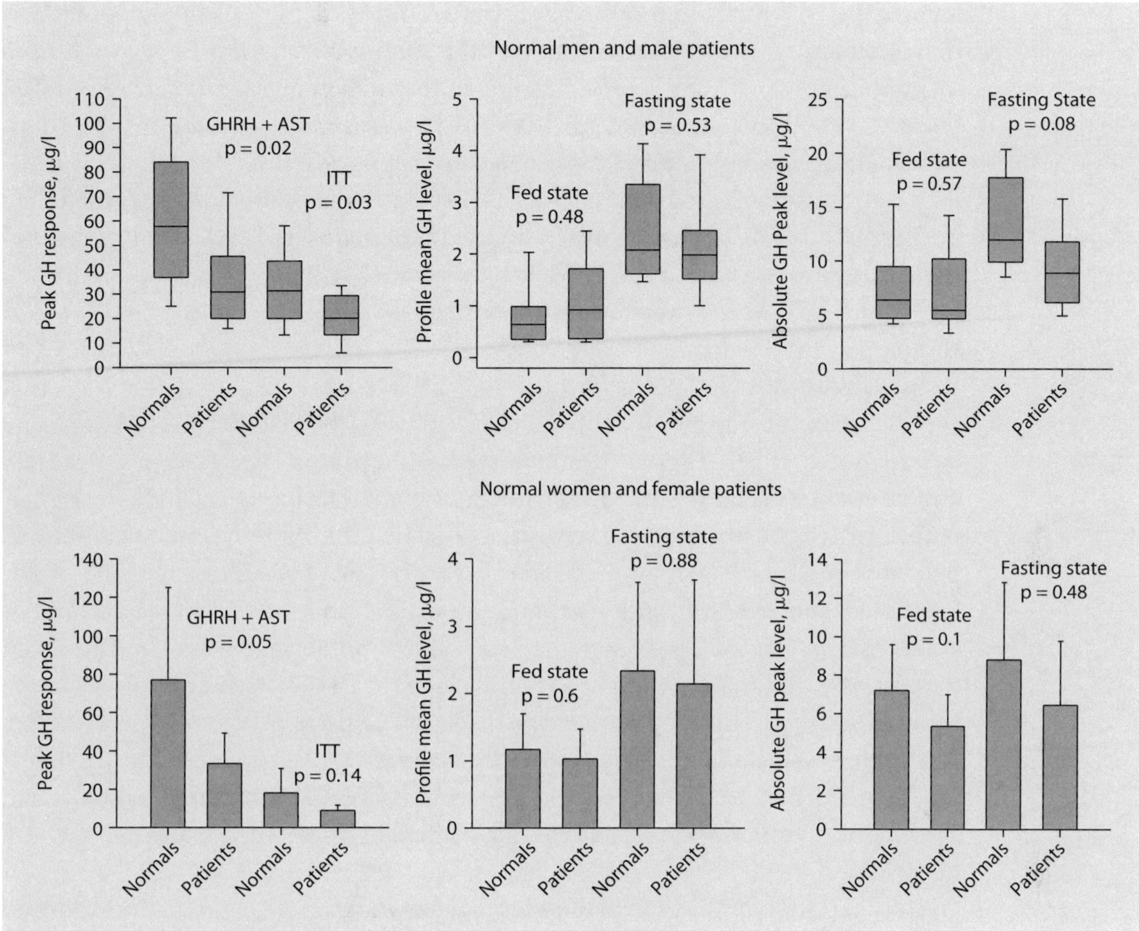

Fig. 4. Gender-specific comparisons between cranially irradiated patients with normal stimulated peak GH responses and normal controls. The upper panel (for men) shows box and whisker plots, in which the lower boundary of the box indicates the 25th percentile, a line within the box marks the median, and the upper boundary of the box indicates the 75th percentile. Error bars above and below the box indicate the 90th and 10th percentiles. In the lower panel (for women), the upper boundary of the box indicates the mean and the error bar indicates 1 SD above the mean. Note the marked reduction in the stimulated GH responses (maximal reserve) in the light of preserved physiological levels in both the fed and fasting states, though with a trend for lower absolute GH peak levels. Note the marked reduction in ITT responses in women compared with men despite increased physiological GH levels. Reproduced with permission from Darzy et al. [24].

somatotropes and GHRH neurons. In other words, the failure of the GH response to the ITT can occur ahead of any decline in spontaneous GH secretion. This accentuated decline, previously attributed to reduced endogenous GHRH due to hypothalamic dysfunction [26, 27, 38–41] may in fact be a consequence of the combined effect of reduced somatotrope mass plus underlying hypothalamic 'hyperactivity', which limits further stimulation by an ITT. This hypothesis is in agreement with the mechanisms of GH stimulation by the ITT; in addition to inhibiting somatostatin tone, insulin-induced hypoglycaemia causes GHRH release [54–57], meaning that further GHRH release is attenuated if the endogenous GHRH pool is reduced at the outset. In support of this concept, many studies have shown increased spontaneous GH secretion in women [47, 58] mediated by increased hypothalamic agonist activity (increased GHRH release) [59, 60], yet the GH responses to an ITT are reduced by as much as 50% and can be subnormal [24, 42, 61–63]; with similar or even increased GH responses to the GHRH+AST compared with normal men [24, 60, 64].

In addition, how can the discordance between the ITT and the AST that appears to mimic, to some extent, that seen between the ITT and the GHRH+AST be explained? It is accepted that increased endogenous GHRH release leads to an increase in somatostatin tone mediated by a paracrine effect [58]. Arginine-induced GH release is believed to be mediated by inhibition of somatostatin tone, but only in the presence of endogenous GHRH [55, 57]. Thus, reversal of the 'increased' somatostatin tone with arginine in the presence of increased endogenous GHRH would be predicted to result in more exaggerated GH responses that may be discordant with the GH responses to the ITT when the H-P axis is hyperstimulated. This may explain the discordance between the AST and the ITT seen in normal women and oestrogen-treated men (AST produces more exuberant GH responses than the ITT) [42, 65] as well as in the irradiated patients who show normal responses to the AST in the context of impaired responses to the ITT [42–46].

How do these findings explain what has been described as radiation-induced GH neurosecretory dysfunction (GHNSD)? The first suggestion of GHNSD following H-P axis irradiation arose from the study by Chrousos et al. [46], in which 2 monkeys irradiated with 40 Gy showed impaired spontaneous GH secretion compared to 2 normal controls. GHNSD was proposed in view of the 'normal' peak GH responses to arginine infusion, though the responses to the ITT were diminished. In humans, the notion that radiation might cause GHNSD arose from a number of studies that showed reduced prepubertal and/or pubertal spontaneous GH secretion after cranial irradiation for leukaemia (18–24 Gy); these studies, however, failed to examine stimulated GH secretion to confirm the presence of a neurosecretory defect [66–69]. Whereas, in studies in which stimulated GH secretion was co-examined, the reduction in prepubertal and/or pubertal spontaneous GH secretion after cranial irradiation for leukaemia (18–24 Gy) was associated with a significant reduction in the overall peak GH responses to stimulation tests of the group including the GHRH test despite the normality of the peak responses in individual patients [31, 70–72]. Similarly, a reduction in spontaneous GH secretion in children irradiated for brain tumours (>40 Gy) was associated with blunting of stimulated peak GH responses to the ITT and/or arginine infusion [43, 73] and a 50% reduction in the overall peak GH responses to GHRH, despite the normality of the individual responses in most patients [74]. The results of these studies seem to have led to a general acceptance that radiation-induced GHNSD is probably a real entity. However, these studies failed to demonstrate a pure neurosecretory defect, i.e. an absolutely normal stimulated but reduced spontaneous GH secretion. The erroneous belief that GHNSD exists in irradiated patients was created partly by the definition of normality to a pharmacological test being an all-or-none phenomenon, i.e. threshold effect, rather than the continuum which clearly exists. In children, in whom GH secretion is more critical than it is in adults, failure of the irradiated H-P axis to meet the requirement for increased GH secretion during growth and puberty may be explained by the presence of 'near maximal' activation of a partially damaged H-P axis allowing for no further amplification during puberty; this is in contrast to what has been previously described as GHNSD [66, 67, 69–71, 75]. In support of this explanation, in previous irradiation studies [71, 74], in which children showed normal but reduced overall stimulated GH responses, spontaneous GH secretion was relatively more attenuated and failed to rise during puberty.

Thus, discordance in stimulated GH responses to various stimuli may indicate the presence of partially or fully compensated GHD. Unlike the GHRH+AST, the ITT reflects the functional reserve of the H-P axis and is a much more robust test in the irradiated child; a failed GH response to the ITT, even in the presence of normal GH responses to other tests, is significant as it can predict the need for GH replacement therapy in an individual in whom the already hyperstimulated GH axis is likely to fail or decompensate at a time of increased GH demands, i.e. during growth and puberty. In adults, a failed response to the ITT in isolation may not necessarily reflect GHD while in contrast a failed response to the GHRH+AST almost always indicates GHD.

Abnormalities of Gonadotropin Secretion

Gonadotropin Deficiency

Gonadotropin deficiency is infrequent after a radiation dose to the H-P axis of less than 40 Gy [76, 77]. However, a remarkable increase in incidence is seen following more intensive radiation schedules [8, 11, 14, 15, 78] and in patients irradiated for pituitary tumours [28, 30] with an onset as early as 12 months after radiotherapy. Gonadotropin deficiency provides a spectrum of severity from subtle (subclinical) abnormalities in secretion, detected only by GnRH testing, to severe impairment associated with diminished circulating sex hormone levels. Although abnormalities in LH/FSH secretion can be demonstrated on dynamic testing, sometimes as early as 1 month following high dose irradiation [15], clinically significant gonadotropin deficiency is usually a late complication with a cumulative incidence of 20–50% after long-term follow-up, making it the second most common anterior pituitary hormone deficit in many series, whether radiation was administered in childhood or adult life [4, 8, 11, 14, 78].

The pattern of LH/FSH responses to GnRH testing may reveal the predominant site of radiation damage, pituitary vs. hypothalamic. Lam et al. [11, 22] demonstrated a progressive decrease in the stimulated but not basal LH level 1, 2, 3, 4 and 5 years after irradiation, whereas basal and stimulated FSH level increased after irradiation and were significantly higher than pre-treatment values at 1 year. After the first year, there was a tendency for both basal and stimulated FSH levels to fall with increasing time since radiotherapy. The mean integrated FSH responses to GnRH stimulation at 3, 4 and 5 years were significantly lower than the mean value at 1 year. The authors suggested that the fall in serum LH but rise in serum FSH in the first year following radiation is due to a radiation-induced decrease in the pulse frequency of hypothalamic GnRH secretion while the progressive decrease in secretion of both LH and FSH after the first year is in keeping with a progressive reduction in hypothalamic GnRH pulse amplitude. In agreement with these conclusions, repeated intermittent infusion of GnRH may restore pituitary responsiveness and therefore differentiate between primary and secondary pituitary atrophy [79] and with prolonged treatment there is the potential for restoring gonadal function and fertility [80].

Precocious or Early Puberty

Radiation doses of <50 Gy may, paradoxically, cause premature activation of the H-P-gonadal axis resulting in early or precocious puberty [81–84]. At low radiation doses such as those used for prophylactic (18–24 Gy) cranial irradiation for acute lymphoblastic leukaemia, precocious puberty occurs almost exclusively in girls [82, 85]. With higher radiation doses (25–50 Gy), however, precocious puberty affects both sexes equally. Ogilvy-Stuart et al. [83] demonstrated that the mean chronological age at the onset of puberty following irradiation for brain tumours (25–50 Gy) was 8.5 years in girls and 9.2 years in boys plus 0.29 year for every year of age at the time of irradiation (fig. 5). In a more recent study, Lannering et al. [84] also showed that boys who received high doses of irradiation for brain tumours entered puberty at a median age of 10.5 years compared to an average age for Swedish boys of 12.4 years; again emphasising the disappearance of sexual dichotomy with higher radiation doses. This is frankly abnormal in the context of GHD, which is often associated with a delay in the onset of puberty.

The mechanism for early puberty after irradiation is likely to be related to the disinhibition of cortical influences on the hypothalamus. Puberty proceeds

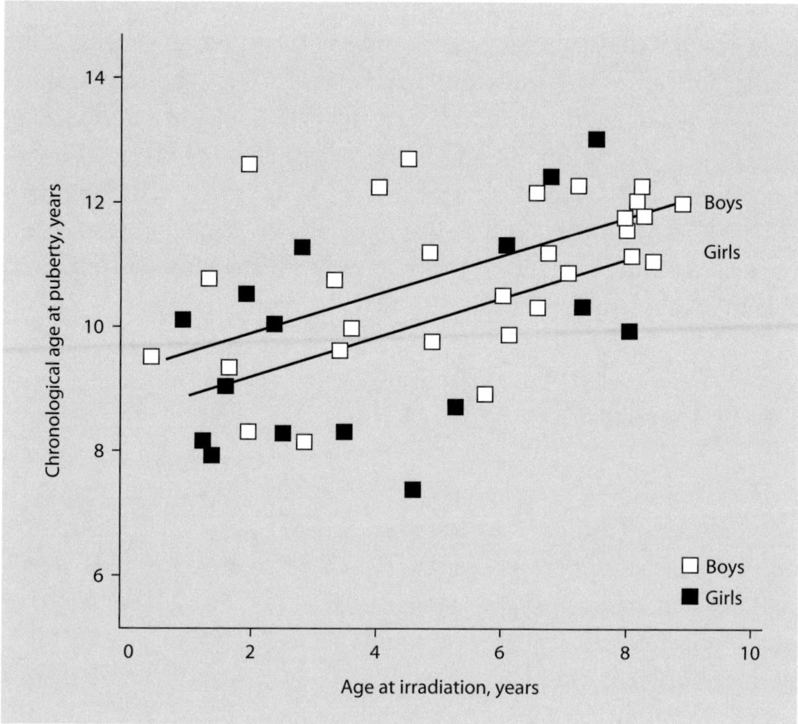

Fig. 5. Estimated and fitted chronological ages at the onset of puberty for age at irradiation. Reproduced with permission from Ogilvy-Stuart et al. [83].

through the increased frequency and amplitude of GnRH pulsatile secretion by the hypothalamus. The clinical observations in humans of radiation dose-dependency of abnormalities in gonadotropin secretion have been confirmed in an animal model. Roth et al. [86] selectively irradiated the H-P region of infantile or juvenile female rats with a single dose of 4, 5, 6, 9 or 2 × 9 Gy. High radiation doses (9 Gy or more) caused retardation of sexual maturation, lower gonadotropin levels and growth retardation associated with GHD, whereas low radiation doses (5 or 6 Gy) led to accelerated onset of puberty as well as elevated LH and estradiol levels in 20% of infantile rats but not the older (juvenile) rats suggesting, in addition, age dependency for the premature activation of the hypothalamic GnRH-pulse generator. The authors also showed that, in animals irradiated with 5 Gy, the release rates of the inhibitory neurotransmitter γ-aminobutyric-acid (GABA) from hypothalamic explants were significantly lower and the GnRH expression in the hypothalamic pre-optic area was significantly higher than in controls [87]. They postulated that radiation-induced precocious puberty might be caused by damage to inhibitory GABAergic neurons leading to disinhibition and premature activation of GnRH neurons.

The outcome of precocious puberty is usually worse in irradiated children as GHD is almost always present leading to attenuation of the pubertal growth spurt resulting in a further loss of growth potential. Furthermore, the window of opportunity offered by GH replacement is reduced in the GH-deficient child who is already pubertal. Thus, the addition of GnRH analogue therapy to GH therapy to halt pubertal progression and delay epiphyseal closure in order to extend the time available for GH to promote linear growth has been shown to be beneficial, but at the expense of exacerbating skeletal disproportion in those who had impaired spinal growth due to spinal irradiation [88, 89].

Abnormalities of ACTH Secretion

The H-P-adrenal axis appears to be relatively radioresistant in patients irradiated for non-pituitary disorders. Clinically apparent ACTH deficiency is uncommon; it occurs in around 3% of patients receiving a total radiation dose to the H-P axis of <50 Gy [8, 21] and it is virtually unreported after TBI [17, 18]. Higher rates of ACTH deficiency were recently reported in adults irradiated after age 16 years (21%), but many had borderline subnormal results [4]. In contrast, the frequency of ACTH deficiency is significantly increased following radiotherapy for non-pituitary brain tumours with doses of >50 Gy with reported rates of 27–35% up to 15 years after irradiation. In most reported cases, however, ACTH deficiency was partial and only a few patients needed regular hydrocortisone replacement because of symptoms of hypocortisolism [8, 11, 14]. A more dramatic increase with incidence rates of 31–60% is seen in patients conventionally irradiated for pituitary tumours [28, 30].

It has been suggested that subtle ACTH deficiency is more frequent following irradiation for brain tumours and this can be demonstrated by reduced 11-deoxycortisol (compound S) responses to metyrapone testing [8, 90]. However, the prevalence of subtle changes in ACTH secretion is dependent upon the interpretation of the metyrapone test results. From a clinical perspective, significant as opposed to subtle abnormalities in ACTH secretion are unlikely to be missed by the ITT, which remains the 'gold standard'. If the ITT is contraindicated, alternative tests like glucagon and synacthen may be considered.

In an attempt to find out if radiation-induced ACTH neurosecretory dysfunction exists, the authors [91] studied spontaneous cortisol secretion by 20-min sampling for 24 h in the fed as well as in the last 24 of a 33-hour fast in 34 adult cancer survivors with normal individual and overall cortisol responses to insulin-induced hypoglycaemia. Paradoxically the study revealed activation of the CRH-ACTH-adrenal axis manifested by a parallel significant increase in mean 24-hour circulating cortisol levels (by 14%) and cortisol production rates (by 20%) without

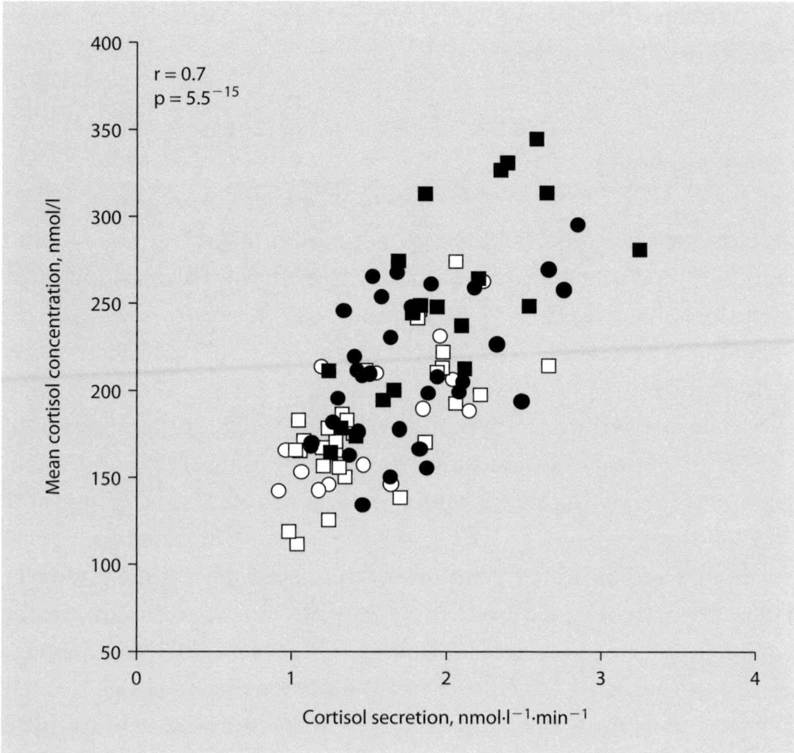

Fig. 6. Cortisol concentrations and total cortisol secretion rates in normal controls and cranially irradiated adult cancer survivors with normal peak cortisol responses to insulin-induced hypoglycaemnia. ● = Patients fed; ■ = patients fasted; ○ = normals fed; □ = normals fasted. Note the shift to the right and upwards in the patients' values. Reproduced with permission from Darzy and Shalet [91].

any changes in cortisol half life, overall secretory pattern or diurnal rhythmicity compared with matched controls (fig. 6). It is speculated that chronic stress associated with the poor quality of life and long-term disabilities from cancer treatment may play a role in this phenomenon. In addition, direct effects of radiation may lead to proactivation of the H-P-adrenal axis through a variety of mechanisms, including radiation-induced CNS inflammation with increased inflammatory and pro-inflammatory cytokines, such as the interleukins, interferons, and tumour necrosis factors, that are known to stimulate CRH release, as well as a radiation-induced reduction in the inhibitory neurotransmitter-GABA that normally inhibits CRH release. With more intensive irradiation and longer post-irradiation periods, the extent of the damage to the CRH neurons and/or /ACTH-secreting cells and the degree of the axis activation will determine the final CRH-ACTH-cortisol secretory status. It is likely that activation of the H-P-adrenal axis is beneficial in reducing the inflammatory and damaging effects of radiation on the brain, but potentially, it could contribute to the development of the metabolic syndrome and osteoporosis in cancer survivors [91].

Abnormalities of TSH Secretion

The H-P-thyroid axis appears to be the least vulnerable to radiation damage and highly dose-dependent [8, 10, 11]. Frank secondary hypothyroidism has not been described following prophylactic (18–24 Gy) cranial irradiation or TBI [17, 18, 92–94] and the incidence of TSH deficiency remains as low as 3–6% in survivors of non-pituitary brain tumours [21, 95]. Patients irradiated during adulthood were reported to have 9% rate of secondary hypothyroidism [4]. A higher incidence of overt secondary hypothyroidism is noted in patients with pituitary tumours [28, 30], but more frequently following intensive irradiation schedules utilising doses of >50 Gy [8, 11, 13–15].

Abnormalities in the dynamics of basal and stimulated TSH secretion, frequently seen in patients with overt central hypothyroidism, are common in euthyroid cancer survivors. Increased basal and stimulated TSH levels and hypothalamic patterns of TSH response during a TRH test in the presence of normal free T4 levels have been reported as soon as 12 months after irradiation [11] and in those followed long-term [23, 96, 97]. The increase in basal and stimulated TSH levels in euthyroid adult cancer survivors has been attributed to a variety of factors. The most important of these are subclinical thyroid dysfunction due to direct thyroid irradiation during cranio-spinal radiotherapy or TBI, especially in the presence of GHD, and scattered irradiation during cranial irradiation alone [97] (fig. 7).

It has been claimed that the presence of a hypothalamic TSH response to a TRH test and/or diminished nocturnal TSH surge despite a normal free T4 level may imply a diagnosis of so-called 'hidden' central hypothyroidism in a substantial proportion of irradiated children [23]. In a recent study by the authors [97], however, it was demonstrated that the loss of nocturnal TSH surge seen in about 20% of 37 euthyroid adult cancer survivors did not reflect a genuine loss of diurnal rhythm, but simply occurred as a result of a physiological shift in the timing of the peak TSH (acrophase) and/or the nadir TSH levels to outside the recommended sampling times (for the nocturnal surge) of 22.00–04.00 h and 14.00–18.00 h, respectively; thereby potentially leading to an erroneous diagnosis of 'hidden' central hypothyroidism. The normality of free T4 levels and the wide discrepancy between the high rate (30%) of these TSH abnormalities and the very low rate of overt secondary hypothyroidism (3–9%) after prolonged periods of post-irradiation follow-up strongly suggest that, in the vast majority of patients, these abnormalities in TSH dynamics represent subtle functional disturbances in the H-P axis rather than genuine pathology that may progress with time.

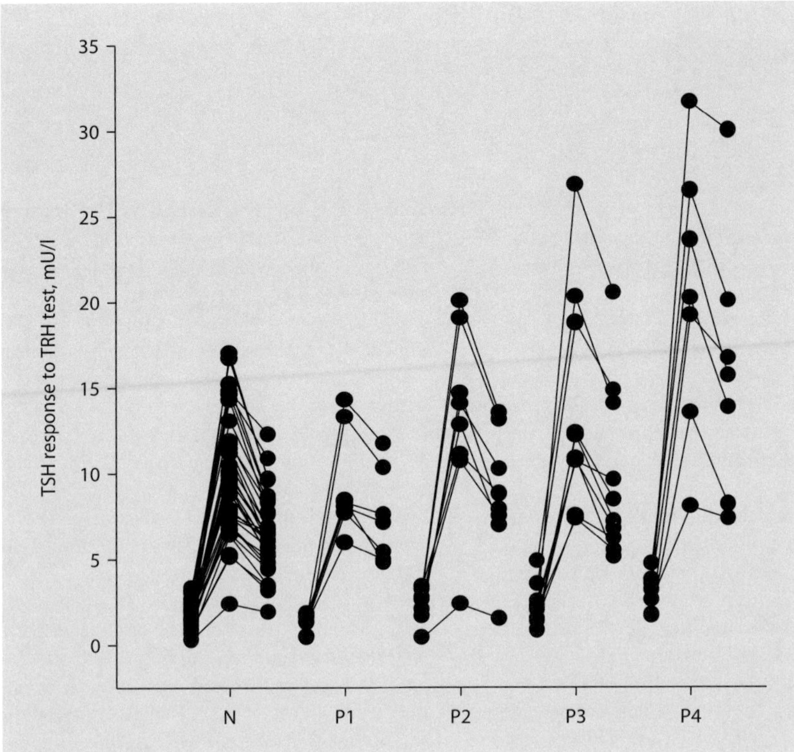

Fig. 7. Individual TSH responses (at 0, 20 and 60 min) to TRH stimulation test in normal controls and cranially irradiated euthyroid adult cancer survivors. CIR = Cranial irradiation; CSI = craniospinal irradiation. Note the impact of spinal irradiation and that of GH deficiency (GHD) or GH insufficiency (GHI) on the basal and stimulated TSH levels. N = Normals; P1 = CIR patients without GHD; P2 = CSI patients without GHD; P3 = CSI patients with GHI; P4 = CSI patients with GHD. Reproduced with permission from Darzy and Shalet [97].

Abnormalities of Prolactin Secretion

Radiation-induced hyperprolactinaemia, due to a reduction in the inhibitory neurotransmitter dopamine, has been described in both sexes and all age groups but is most frequently encountered in the adult female with radiation doses of >40 Gy. In these patients, a mild to modest elevation in prolactin level is noticed in 20–50% [4, 8, 11, 14, 28] compared with less than 5% in children [78] and after low radiation doses [18]. Radiation-induced hyperprolactinaemia is not associated with significant biological impact in the vast majority of patients. Occasionally, it may be of sufficient severity to impair gonadotropin secretion and cause pubertal delay or arrest in children, decreased libido and impotence in adult males and galactorrhoea and/or amenorrhoea in women [14]. A gradual decline in the elevated prolactin level may occur with time and can normalise in some patients. This may reflect time-dependent slowly evolving direct radiation-induced damage to the pituitary lactotrope [28].

References

1 Withers HR: Biology of radiation oncology; in Tobias JS, Thomas PRM (eds): Current Radiation Oncology. London, Edward Arnold 1994, vol 1, pp 5–23.

2 Schmiegelow M, Lassen S, Poulsen HS, Feldt-Rasmussen U, Schmiegelow K, Hertz H, Muller J: Cranial radiotherapy of childhood brain tumours: growth hormone deficiency and its relation to the biological effective dose of irradiation in a large population based study. Clin Endocrinol 2000;53: 191–197.

3 Darzy KH, Aimaretti G, Wieringa G, Gattamaneni HR, Ghigo E, Shalet SM: The usefulness of the combined growth hormone (GH)-releasing hormone and arginine stimulation test in the diagnosis of radiation-induced GH deficiency is dependent on the post-irradiation time interval. J Clin Endocrinol Metab 2003;88:95–102.

4 Agha A, Sherlock M, Brennan S, O'Connor SA, O'Sullivan E, Rogers B, Faul C, Rawluk D, Tormey W, Thompson CJ: Hypothalamic-pituitary dysfunction after irradiation of nonpituitary brain tumors in adults. J Clin Endocrinol Metab 2005; 90:6355–6360.

5 Chieng PU, Huang TS, Chang CC, Chong PN, Tien RD, Su CT: Reduced hypothalamic blood flow after radiation treatment of nasopharyngeal cancer: SPECT studies in 34 patients. Am J Neuroradiol 1991;12:661–665.

6 Hochberg Z, Kuten A, Hertz P, Tatcher M, Kedar A, Benderly A: The effect of single-dose radiation on cell survival and growth hormone secretion by rat anterior pituitary cells. Radiat Res 1983;94: 508–512.

7 Robinson IC, Fairhall KM, Hendry JH, Shalet SM: Differential radiosensitivity of hypothalamo-pituitary function in the young adult rat. J Endocrinol 2001;169:519–526.

8 Constine LS, Woolf PD, Cann D, Mick G, McCormick K, Raubertas RF, Rubin P: Hypothalamic-pituitary dysfunction after radiation for brain tumors. N Engl J Med 1993;328:87–94.

9 Clayton PE, Shalet SM: Dose dependency of time of onset of radiation-induced growth hormone deficiency. J Pediatr 1991;118:226–228.

10 Littley MD, Shalet SM, Beardwell CG, Robinson EL, Sutton ML: Radiation-induced hypopituitarism is dose-dependent. Clin Endocrinol Oxf 1989;31:363–373.

11 Lam KS, Tse VK, Wang C, Yeung RT, Ho JH: Effects of cranial irradiation on hypothalamic-pituitary function – a 5-year longitudinal study in patients with nasopharyngeal carcinoma. Q J Med 1991;78:165–176.

12 Duffner PK, Cohen ME, Voorhess ML, MacGillivray MH, Brecher ML, Panahon A, Gilani BB: Long-term effects of cranial irradiation on endocrine function in children with brain tumors. A prospective study. Cancer 1985;56: 2189–2193.

13 Pai HH, Thornton A, Katznelson L, Finkelstein DM, Adams JA, Fullerton BC, Loeffler JS, Leibsch NJ, Klibanski A, Munzenrider JE: Hypothalamic/pituitary function following high-dose conformal radiotherapy to the base of skull: demonstration of a dose-effect relationship using dose-volume histogram analysis. J Radiat Oncol Biol Phys 2001;49:1079–1092.

14 Samaan NA, Vieto R, Schultz PN, Maor M, Meoz RT, Sampiere VA, Cangir A, Ried HL, Jesse RH Jr: Hypothalamic, pituitary and thyroid dysfunction after radiotherapy to the head and neck. Int J Radiat Oncol Biol Phys 1982;8:1857–1867.

15 Chen MS, Lin FJ, Huang MJ, Wang PW, Tang S, Leung WM, Leung W: Prospective hormone study of hypothalamic-pituitary function in patients with nasopharyngeal carcinoma after high dose irradiation. Jpn J Clin Oncol 1989;19: 265–270.

16 Sham J, Choy D, Kwong PW, Cheng AC, Kwong DL, Yau CC, Wan KY, Au GK: Radiotherapy for nasopharyngeal carcinoma: shielding the pituitary may improve therapeutic ratio. Int J Radiat Oncol Biol Phys 1994;29:699–704.

17 Ogilvy-Stuart AL, Clark DJ, Wallace WH, Gibson BE, Stevens RF, Shalet SM, Donaldson MD: Endocrine deficit after fractionated total body irradiation. Arch Dis Child 1992;67:1107–1110.

18 Littley MD, Shalet SM, Morgenstern GR, Deakin DP: Endocrine and reproductive dysfunction following fractionated total body irradiation in adults. Q J Med 1991;78:265–274.

19 Brauner R, Czernichow P, Rappaport R: Greater susceptibility to hypothalamopituitary irradiation in younger children with acute lymphoblastic leukemia. J Pediatr 1986;108:332.

20 Samaan NA, Schultz PN, Yang KP, Vassilopoulou-Sellin R, Maor MH, Cangir A, Goepfert H: Endocrine complications after radiotherapy for tumors of the head and neck. J Lab Clin Med 1987;109:364–372.

21 Livesey EA, Hindmarsh PC, Brook CG, Whitton AC, Bloom HJ, Tobias JS, Godlee JN, Britton J: Endocrine disorders following treatment of childhood brain tumours. Br J Cancer 1990;61:622–625.

22 Lam KS, Tse VK, Wang C, Yeung RT, Ma JT, Ho JH: Early effects of cranial irradiation on hypothalamic-pituitary function. J Clin Endocrinol Metab 1987;64:418–424.

23 Rose SR, Lustig RH, Pitukcheewanont P, Broome DC, Burghen GA, Li H, Hudson MM, Kun LE, Heideman RL: Diagnosis of hidden central hypothyroidism in survivors of childhood cancer. J Clin Endocrinol Metab 1999;84:4472–4479.

24 Darzy KH, Pezzoli SS, Thorner MO, Shalet SM: Cranial irradiation and growth hormone neurosecretory dysfunction: a critical appraisal. J Clin Endocrinol Metab 2007;92:1666–1672.

25 Marekova M, Cap J, Vokurkova D, Vavrova J, Cerman J: Effect of therapeutic doses of ionising radiation on the somatomammotroph pituitary cell line, GH3. Endocr J 2003;50:621–628.

26 Schmiegelow M, Lassen S, Poulsen HS, Feldt-Rasmussen U, Schmiegelow K, Hertz H, Muller J: Growth hormone response to a growth hormone-releasing hormone stimulation test in a population-based study following cranial irradiation of childhood brain tumors. Horm Res 2000;54:53–59.

27 Achermann JC, Brook CG, Hindmarsh PC: The GH response to low-dose bolus growth hormone-releasing hormone (GHRH(1–29)NH2) is attenuated in patients with longstanding post-irradiation GH insufficiency. Eur J Endocrinol 2000;142:359–364.

28 Littley MD, Shalet SM, Beardwell CG, Ahmed SR, Applegate G, Sutton ML: Hypopituitarism following external radiotherapy for pituitary tumours in adults. Q J Med 1989;70:145–160.

29 Nishioka H, Ito H, Haraoka J, Hirano A: Histological changes in the hypofunctional pituitary gland following conventional radiotherapy for adenoma. Histopathology 2001;38:561–566.

30 Rush S, Cooper PR: Symptom resolution, tumor control, and side effects following postoperative radiotherapy for pituitary macroadenomas. Int J Radiat Oncol Biol Phys 1997;37:1031–1034.

31 Costin G: Effects of low-dose cranial radiation on growth hormone secretory dynamics and hypothalamic-pituitary function. Am J Dis Child 1988;142:847–852.

32 Brennan BM, Rahim A, Mackie EM, Eden OB, Shalet SM: Growth hormone status in adults treated for acute lymphoblastic leukaemia in childhood. Clin Endocrinol (Oxf) 1998;48:777–783.

33 Giorgiani G, Bozzola M, Locatelli F, Picco P, Zecca M, Cisternino M, Dallorso S, Bonetti F, Dini G, Borrone C, Regazzi MB, et al: Role of busulfan and total body irradiation on growth of prepubertal children receiving bone marrow transplantation and results of treatment with recombinant human growth hormone. Blood 1995;86:825–831.

34 Brauner R, Adan L, Souberbielle JC, Esperou H, Michon J, Devergie A, Gluckman E, Zucker JM: Contribution of growth hormone deficiency to the growth failure that follows bone marrow transplantation. J Pediatr 1997;130:785–792.

35 Shalet SM, Beardwell CG, Morris-Jones PH, Pearson D: Pituitary function after treatment of intracranial tumours in children. Lancet 1975;2:104–107.

36 Gleeson HK, Gattamaneni HR, Smethurst L, Brennan BM, Shalet SM: Reassessment of growth hormone status is required at final height in children treated with growth hormone replacement after radiation therapy. J Clin Endocrinol Metab 2004;89:662–666.

37 Shalet SM, Toogood AA, Rahim A, Brennan BMD: The diagnosis of growth hormone deficiency in children and adults. Endocr Rev 1998;19:203–223.

38 Lustig RH, Schriock EA, Kaplan SL, Grumbach MM: Effect of growth hormone-releasing factor on growth hormone release in children with radiation-induced growth hormone deficiency. Pediatrics 1985;76:274–279.

39 Grossman A, Savage MO, Blacklay A, Ross RM, Plowman PN, Preece MA, Coy DH, Besser GM: The use of growth hormone-releasing hormone in the diagnosis and treatment of short stature. Horm Res 1985;22:52–57.

40 Oberfield SE, Kirkland JL, Frantz A, Allen JC, Levine LS: Growth hormone response to GRF 1–44 in children following cranial irradiation for central nervous system tumors. Am J Pediatr Hematol Oncol 1987;9:233–238.

41 Crosnier H, Brauner R, Rappaport R: Growth hormone response to growth hormone-releasing hormone (hp GHRH1–44) as an index of growth hormone secretory dysfunction after prophylactic cranial irradiation for acute lymphoblastic leukemia (24 grays). Acta Paediatr Scand 1988;77: 681–687.
42 Lissett CA, Saleem S, Rahim A, Brennan BM, Shalet SM: The impact of irradiation on growth hormone responsiveness to provocative agents is stimulus dependent: results in 161 individuals with radiation damage to the somatotropic axis. J Clin Endocrinol Metab 2001;86:663–668.
43 Ahmed SR, Shalet SM, Beardwell CG: The effects of cranial irradiation on growth hormone secretion. Acta Paediatr Scand 1986;75:255–260.
44 Romshe CA, Zipf WB, Miser A, Miser J, Sotos JF, Newton WA: Evaluation of growth hormone release and human growth hormone treatment in children with cranial irradiation-associated short stature. J Pediatr 1984;104:177–181.
45 Dickinson WP, Berry DH, Dickinson L, Irvin M, Schedewie H, Fiser RH, Elders MJ: Differential effects of cranial radiation on growth hormone response to arginine and insulin infusion. J Pediatr 1978;92:754–757.
46 Chrousos GP, Poplack D, Brown T, O'Neill D, Schwade J, Bercu BB: Effects of cranial radiation on hypothalamic-adenohypophyseal function: abnormal growth hormone secretory dynamics. J Clin Endocrinol Metab 1982;54:1135–1139.
47 Darzy K, Pezzoli S, Thorner M, Shalet S: The dynamics of GH secretion in adult cancer survivors with severe GH deficiency acquired following brain irradiation in childhood for non-pituitary brain tumors: evidence for preserved pulsatility and diurnal variation with increased secretory disorderliness. J Clin Endocrinol Metab 2005;90: 2794–2803.
48 Jessup SK, Malow BA, Symons KV, Barkan AL: Blockade of endogenous growth hormone-releasing hormone receptors dissociates nocturnal growth hormone secretion and slow-wave sleep. Eur J Endocrinol 2004;151:561–566.
49 Ocampo-Lim B, Guo W, DeMott-Friberg R, Barkan AL, Jaffe CA: Nocturnal growth hormone (GH) secretion is eliminated by infusion of GH-releasing hormone antagonist. J Clin Endocrinol Metab 1996;81:4396–4399.
50 Wehrenberg WB, Brazeau P, Luben R, Bohlen P, Guillemin R: Inhibition of the pulsatile secretion of growth hormone by monoclonal antibodies to the hypothalamic growth hormone releasing factor (GRF). Endocrinology. 1982;111:2147–2148.
51 Sklar CA, Constine LS: Chronic neuroendocrinological sequelae of radiation therapy. Int J Radiat Oncol Biol Phys 1995;31:1113–1121.
52 Paakko E, Talvensaari K, Pyhtinen J, Lanning M: Decreased pituitary gland height after radiation treatment to the hypothalamic-pituitary axis evaluated by MR. AJNR Am J Neuroradiol 1994; 15:537–541.
53 Darzy KH, Thorner MO, Shalet SM: Cranially irradiated adult cancer survivors may have normal spontaneous GH secretion in the presence of discordant peak GH responses to stimulation tests (compensated GH deficiency). Clin Endocrinol 2008; e-pub ahead of print.
54 Kashio Y, Chihara K, Kita T, Okimura Y, Sato M, Kadowaki S, Fujita T: Effect of oral glucose administration on plasma growth hormone-releasing hormone (GHRH)-like immunoreactivity levels in normal subjects and patients with idiopathic GH deficiency: evidence that GHRH is released not only from the hypothalamus but also from extrahypothalamic tissue. J Clin Endocrinol Metab 1987;64:92–97.
55 Masuda A, Shibasaki T, Hotta M, Yamauchi N, Ling N, Demura H, Shizume K: Insulin-induced hypoglycemia, L-dopa and arginine stimulate GH secretion through different mechanisms in man. Regul Pept 1990;31:53–64.
56 Koppeschaar HP, ten Horn CD, Thijssen JH, Page MD, Dieguez C, Scanlon MF: Differential effects of arginine on growth hormone releasing hormone and insulin induced growth hormone secretion. Clin Endocrinol Oxf 1992;36:487–490.
57 Hanew K, Utsumi A: The role of endogenous GHRH in arginine-, insulin-, clonidine- and L-dopa-induced GH release in normal subjects. Eur J Endocrinol 2002;146:197–202.
58 Giustina A, Veldhuis JD: Pathophysiology of the neuroregulation of growth hormone secretion in experimental animals and the human. Endocr Rev 1998;19:717–797.
59 Veldhuis JD, Farhy L, Weltman AL, Kuipers J, Weltman J, Wideman L: Gender modulates sequential suppression and recovery of pulsatile growth hormone secretion by physiological feedback signals in young adults. J Clin Endocrinol Metab 2005;90:2874–2881.
60 Soares-Welch C, Farhy L, Mielke KL, Mahmud FH, Miles JM, Bowers CY, Veldhuis JD: Complementary secretagogue pairs unmask prominent gender-related contrasts in mechanisms of growth hormone pulse renewal in young adults. J Clin Endocrinol Metab 2005;90:2225–2232.

61 Hoeck HC, Vestergaard P, Jakobsen PE, Laurberg P: Test of growth hormone secretion in adults: poor reproducibility of the insulin tolerance test. Eur J Endocrinol 1995;133:305–312.
62 Diamond MP, Jones T, Caprio S, Hallarman L, Diamond MC, Addabbo M, Tamborlane WV, Sherwin RS: Gender influences counterregulatory hormone responses to hypoglycemia. Metabolism 1993;42:1568–1572.
63 Osterman PO, Wide L: The insulin tolerance test after pre-treatment with dexamethasone. Acta Endocrinol Copenh 1976;83:341–356.
64 Biller BM, Samuels MH, Zagar A, Cook DM, Arafah BM, Bonert V, Stavrou S, Kleinberg DL, Chipman JJ, Hartman ML: Sensitivity and specificity of six tests for the diagnosis of adult GH deficiency. J Clin Endocrinol Metab 2002;87: 2067–2079.
65 Merimee TJ, Rabinowtitz D, Fineberg SE: Arginine-initiated release of human growth hormone. Factors modifying the response in normal man. N Engl J Med 1969;280:1434–1438.
66 Blatt J, Lee P, Suttner J, Finegold D: Pulsatile growth hormone secretion in children with acute lymphoblastic leukemia after 1800 cGy cranial radiation. Int J Radiat Oncol Biol Phys 1988;15: 1001–1006.
67 Crowne EC, Moore C, Wallace WH, Ogilvy-Stuart AL, Addison GM, Morris-Jones PH, Shalet SM: A novel variant of growth hormone (GH) insufficiency following low dose cranial irradiation. Clin Endocrinol (Oxf) 1992;36:59–68.
67 Stubberfield TG, Byrne GC, Jones TW: Growth and growth hormone secretion after treatment for acute lymphoblastic leukemia in childhood. 18-Gy versus 24-Gy cranial irradiation. J Pediatr Hematol Oncol 1995;17:167–171.
69 Lannering B, Rosberg S, Marky I, Moell C, Albertsson-Wikland K: Reduced growth hormone secretion with maintained periodicity following cranial irradiation in children with acute lymphoblastic leukaemia. Clin Endocrinol (Oxf) 1995;42:153–159.
70 Blatt J, Bercu BB, Gillin JC, Mendelson WB, Poplack DG: Reduced pulsatile growth hormone secretion in children after therapy for acute lymphoblastic leukemia. J Pediatr 1984;104:182–186.
71 Moell C, Garwicz S, Westgren U, Wiebe T, Albertsson-Wikland K: Suppressed spontaneous secretion of growth hormone in girls after treatment for acute lymphoblastic leukaemia. Arch Dis Child 1989;64:252–258.
72 Ryalls M, Spoudeas HA, Hindmarsh PC, Matthews DR, Tait DM, Meller ST, Brook CG: Short-term endocrine consequences of total body irradiation and bone marrow transplantation in children treated for leukemia. J Endocrinol 1993; 136:331–338.
73 Spoudeas HA, Hindmarsh PC, Matthews DR, Brook CG: Evolution of growth hormone neurosecretory disturbance after cranial irradiation for childhood brain tumours: a prospective study. J Endocrinol 1996;150:329–342.
74 Lannering B, Albertsson-Wikland K: Growth hormone release in children after cranial irradiation. Horm Res 1987;27:13–22.
75 Moell C: Disturbed pubertal growth in girls after acute leukaemia: a relative growth hormone insufficiency with late presentation. Acta Paediatr Scand Suppl 1988;343:162–166.
76 Pasqualini T, Escobar ME, Domene H, Muriel FS, Pavlovsky S, Rivarola MA: Evaluation of gonadal function following long-term treatment for acute lymphoblastic leukemia in girls. Am J Pediatr Hematol Oncol 1987;9:15–22.
77 Sanders JE, Buckner CD, Leonard JM, Sullivan KM, Witherspoon RP, Deeg HJ, Storb R, Thomas ED: Late effects on gonadal function of cyclophosphamide, total-body irradiation, and marrow transplantation. Transplantation 1983;36: 252–255.
78 Rappaport R, Brauner R, Czernichow P, Thibaud E, Renier D, Zucker JM, Lemerle J: Effect of hypothalamic and pituitary irradiation on pubertal development in children with cranial tumors. J Clin Endocrinol Metab 1982;54:1164–1168.
79 Yoshimoto Y, Moridera K, Imura H: Restoration of normal pituitary gonadotropin reserve by administration of luteinizing-hormone-releasing hormone in patients with hypogonadotropic hypogonadism. N Engl J Med 1975;292:242–245.
80 Hall JE, Martin KA, Whitney HA, Landy H, Crowley WF Jr: Potential for fertility with replacement of hypothalamic gonadotropin-releasing hormone in long term female survivors of cranial tumors. J Clin Endocrinol Metab 1994;79:1166–1172.
81 Brauner R, Rappaport R: Precocious puberty secondary to cranial irradiation for tumors distant from the hypothalamo-pituitary area. Horm Res 1985;22:78–82.
82 Leiper AD, Stanhope R, Kitching P, Chessells JM: Precocious and premature puberty associated with treatment of acute lymphoblastic leukaemia. Arch Dis Child 1987;62:1107–1112.

83 Ogilvy-Stuart AL, Clayton PE, Shalet SM: Cranial irradiation and early puberty. J Clin Endocrinol Metab 1994;78:1282–1286.
84 Lannering B, Jansson C, Rosberg S, Albertsson-Wikland K: Increased LH and FSH secretion after cranial irradiation in boys. Med Pediatr Oncol 1997;29:280–287.
85 Quigley C, Cowell C, Jimenez M, Burger H, Kirk J, Bergin M, Stevens M, Simpson J, Silink M: Normal or early development of puberty despite gonadal damage in children treated for acute lymphoblastic leukemia. N Engl J Med 1989;321:143–151.
86 Roth C, Schmidberger H, Schaper O, Leonhardt S, Lakomek M, Wuttke W, Jarry H: Cranial irradiation of female rats causes dose-dependent and age-dependent activation or inhibition of pubertal development. Pediatr Res 2000;47:586–591.
87 Roth C, Lakomek M, Schmidberger H, Jarry H: Cranial irradiation induces premature activation of the gonadotropin-releasing-hormone (in German). Klin Pädiatr 2001;213:239–243.
88 Adan L, Sainte-Rose C, Souberbielle JC, Zucker JM, Kalifa C, Brauner R: Adult height after growth hormone (GH) treatment for GH deficiency due to cranial irradiation. Med Pediatr Oncol 2000;34:14–19.
89 Gleeson HK, Stoeter R, Ogilvy-Stuart AL, Gattamaneni HR, Brennan BM, Shalet SM: Improvements in final height over 25 years in growth hormone (GH)-deficient childhood survivors of brain tumors receiving GH replacement. J Clin Endocrinol Metab 2003;88:3682–3689.
90 Rose SR, Lustig RH, Burstein S, Pitukcheewanont P, Broome DC, Burghen GA: Diagnosis of ACTH deficiency. Comparison of overnight metyrapone test to either low-dose or high-dose ACTH test. Horm Res 1999;52:73–79.
91 Darzy KH, Shalet SM: Absence of adrenocorticotropin (ACTH) neurosecretory dysfunction but increased cortisol concentrations and production rates in ACTH-replete adult cancer survivors after cranial irradiation for nonpituitary brain tumors. J Clin Endocrinol Metab 2005;90:5217–5225.
92 Mohn A, Chiarelli F, Di Marzio A, Impicciatore P, Marsico S, Angrilli F: Thyroid function in children treated for acute lymphoblastic leukemia. J Endocrinol Invest 1997;20:215–219.
93 Lando A, Holm K, Nysom K, Rasmussen AK, Feldt-Rasmussen U, Petersen JH, Muller J: Thyroid function in survivors of childhood acute lymphoblastic leukaemia: the significance of prophylactic cranial irradiation. Clin Endocrinol 2001;55:21–25.
94 Carter EP, Leiper AD, Chessells JM, Hurst A: Thyroid function in children after treatment for acute lymphoblastic leukaemia. Arch Dis Child 1989;64:631.
95 Oberfield SE, Sklar C, Allen J, Walker R, Mcelwain M, Papadakis V, Maenza J: Thyroid and gonadal function and growth of long-term survivors of medulloblastoma/PNET; in Green DM, D'Angio GJ (eds): Late Effects of Treatment for Childhood Cancer. New York, Wiley-Liss, 1992, pp 55–62.
96 Schmiegelow M, Feldt-Rasmussen U, Rasmussen AK, Poulsen HS, Muller J: A population-based study of thyroid function after radiotherapy and chemotherapy for a childhood brain tumor. J Clin Endocrinol Metab 2003;88:136–140.
97 Darzy KH, Shalet SM: Circadian and stimulated thyrotropin secretion in cranially irradiated adult cancer survivors. J Clin Endocrinol Metab 2005;90:6490–6497.

Stephen M. Shalet
Professor of Endocrinology
Department of Endocrinology, Christie Hospital NHS Trust
Wilmslow Road, Withington
Manchester M20 4BX (UK)
Tel. +44 161 446 3667, Fax +44 161 446 3772
E-Mail stephen.m.shalet@man.ac.uk

Wallace WHB, Kelnar CJH (eds): Endocrinopathy after Childhood Cancer Treatment.
Endocr Dev. Basel, Karger, 2009, vol 15, pp 25–39

Alterations in Pubertal Timing following Therapy for Childhood Malignancies

Gregory T. Armstrong[a] · Eric J. Chow[b] · Charles A. Sklar[c]

[a]Department of Epidemiology and Cancer Control, St. Jude Children's Research Hospital, Memphis, Tenn., [b]Department of Pediatrics, University of Washington, Seattle, Wash., and [c]Department of Pediatrics, Memorial Sloan-Kettering Cancer Center, New York, N.Y., USA

Abstract

The onset of puberty marks a time of rapid linear growth, sexual development, and transition from childhood to maturity. The diagnosis and treatment of a childhood malignancy prior to the onset of puberty has the potential to profoundly affect the timing and the tempo of puberty. CNS tumors located in the hypothalamic-pituitary (H-P) region, surgical resection in this location, and exposure to CNS radiotherapy are all associated with both precocious and delayed puberty. Also, chemotherapy and radiation can directly damage the gonads, which can result in absent, arrested, or delayed puberty. As a consequence of these alterations of pubertal timing, both male and female survivors of childhood cancer may be at risk of adult short-stature, decreased bone-mineral density, absent or incomplete sexual development, and ultimately, reduced rates of fertility. Appropriate and timely assessment of survivors at high risk of alterations in pubertal development will enable the identification of patients who would benefit from early medical intervention.

The onset of puberty marks a time of rapid linear growth, sexual development, and transition from childhood to maturity. As a result, children experience the appearance of secondary sexual characteristics, the adolescent growth spurt, and the establishment of fertility. This occurs as a consequence of central nervous system (CNS) maturation and release of pituitary gonadotropins resulting in stimulation of gonadal end organs (testis/ovaries) [1]. The diagnosis and treatment of a childhood malignancy prior to the onset of puberty has the potential to profoundly impact the timing and the tempo of puberty. CNS tumors located in the hypothalamic-pituitary (H-P) region, surgical resection in this location, and exposure to CNS radiotherapy are all associated with both precocious and delayed puberty. Also to be considered, chemotherapy and radiation exposure to the gonads can result in premature gonadal failure that may be clinically evident as absent, delayed, or arrested puberty. As a consequence of these alterations of pubertal timing, survivors of childhood cancer may be at risk of adult short stature, decreased bone mineral density, absent or incomplete sexual development and ultimately, reduced rates of fertility. Currently, 80% of children treated for childhood malignancies will become long-term survivors of their cancer [2, 3]. Therefore, understanding which patients are at high risk of alterations in pubertal timing is essential. Appropriate and timely assessment of these patients will allow identification of survivors who would benefit from early medical intervention.

Normal Puberty

The onset of puberty in females is heralded by an increase in height velocity with simultaneous maturation of the glandular and connective tissue of the mammary gland (thelarche). Adrenarche, the growth of pubic and axillary hair, is a phenomenon distinct from breast development as it is largely controlled by androgens secreted by the adrenal gland. Nonetheless, pubic hair development generally parallels breast development. The onset of menses typically correlates with Tanner stage 4 breast development and occurs at an average age of 12.4 years [4]. Several large epidemiologic investigations in the United States, using both representative population samples and large convenience samples, have concluded that a secular trend towards earlier sexual development in females has occurred over the last few decades [5]. Moreover, there appear to be differences between girls of various racial and ethnic backgrounds. For example, non-Hispanic Black girls appear to mature earlier than their Hispanic and Caucasian counterparts [4]. However, while it appears that girls are maturing earlier than they did several decades ago, the age at menarche appears to have changed very little if at all [5]. A recent British study with a more homogeneous population has also shown minimal change in the age of menarche over the past few decades [6]. It has been postulated that this trend to earlier onset of puberty may be related to the recent increase in the rates of childhood obesity.

Across most studies, age at onset of puberty follows a normal distribution with a standard deviation of approximately 1 year. Routinely, children with onset or delay of puberty more than 2 standard deviations from the mean should be considered for medical evaluation of precocious or delayed onset of puberty. For girls, transition from Tanner stage 1 to 2 of breast development is defined by the development of a breast bud and occurs at a mean age of 10 years [7]. Following this standard, females who develop breast buds before age 8 are classified as having precocious puberty, while delayed puberty is defined as no evidence of breast development by age 13.

Among males, the beginning of puberty is marked by an increase in testicular volume followed shortly by the development of pubic hair and growth and maturation of the penis. Finally, peak height velocity occurs between Tanner stages 4 and 5 of genital development. The mean onset of puberty in males is 11 years with limits at 2 standard deviations extending the normal range of onset to 9–14 years of age. Testicular enlargement or other signs of virilization before age 9 are considered precocious. Similarly, a male with no evidence of testicular enlargement by age 14 should be evaluated for delayed onset of puberty. It is important to note that testicular enlargement is largely secondary to growth of the sperm-producing seminiferous tubules, which are very susceptible to damage by various chemotherapeutic agents (e.g. alkylating agents) and external radiation. Thus, for many male cancer survivors, testicular size is not a reliable marker of pubertal maturation as the testes may remain small despite the onset of puberty.

The control mechanisms involved in the timing of the onset of puberty are poorly understood. However, an increase in the pulsatile rate of release of GnRH from the medial basal hypothalamus is the initiating factor for the onset of puberty. In response to this increased rate of release of GnRH, the anterior pituitary releases LH and FSH in a likewise pulsatile manner. The end result is stimulation of the gonads by these gonadotropin pulses, resulting in production and release of gonadal sex steroids. During childhood, the CNS exerts restraint on the hypothalamic GnRH-secreting neurons and pulsatile release of GnRH is suppressed. During CNS maturation, however, these poorly understood restraining forces subside and hypothalamic release of GnRH is reactivated, allowing the normal onset of puberty [1].

Early Puberty

Precocious puberty can occur as a result of either tumor or radiotherapy-induced disruptions of H-P axis regulation of pubertal timing. Precocious puberty can be a presenting symptom of a CNS tumor in both males and females [8, 9]. Among 197 girls and 16 boys who presented with precocious puberty in a British series, 2 girls and 1 boy were subsequently found to have a CNS tumor [9]. In a separate series of 100 children with precocious puberty due to a CNS lesion, 45 had optic pathway gliomas or astrocytomas; 8 presented with precocious puberty, while the other 37 developed symptoms following treatment of their tumor [10]. Optic pathway gliomas, which most commonly present in the anterior half of the optic pathway, are a subgroup of astrocytomas that place a patient at particular risk of early puberty due to their proximity to the H-P axis. Other CNS lesions associated with precocious puberty include benign lesions such as hamartomas and cysts, and more rarely, craniopharyngiomas [10, 11]. Craniopharyngiomas are benign, slow-growing tumors thought to arise from Rathke's pouch (epithelial remnant of the craniopharyngeal duct) [12]. These lesions can all occur in the region of the H-P axis and disrupt hormonal regulation due to direct mass effect and/or hydrocephalus secondary to ventricular system obstruction. The result is an increased risk of early (but also delayed) pubertal onset. Lastly, germ cell tumors, including those arising within and outside the CNS, also can cause precocious puberty, primarily in males, through the production of hCG [13].

Effects of Central Nervous System Radiation

Overall among childhood cancer patients, central precocious puberty occurs most commonly following radiotherapy to the H-P region. Among patients with CNS tumors outside the H-P axis who received radiotherapy (doses 25–72 Gy), both male and female survivors were on average more likely to start puberty earlier (in some reports >1.5 years earlier) compared with population or reference norms [14–16]. Younger age at exposure was also associated with earlier onset of puberty in both sexes [14, 15]. However, cranial radiotherapy doses of 30–40 Gy are also associated with an increased risk of inducing gonadotropin deficiency, resulting in failure of pubertal maturation [17, 18].

Early puberty, at least among girls, has also been seen following exposure to lower doses of cranial radiotherapy given as part of treatment for childhood acute lymphoblastic leukemia (ALL). Historically, even in the absence of detectable CNS leukemia, cranial radiotherapy was used widely to prevent subsequent CNS recurrences. Although cranial radiotherapy has largely been replaced by high dose methotrexate and intrathecal chemotherapy in many current treatment protocols, around 10–15% of ALL patients still receive cranial radiation, usually between 12 and 25 Gy [19]. A report by Quigley et al. [20] in 1989 found that among Australian ALL survivors, 24 Gy cranial radiotherapy was associated with earlier pubertal onset and progression to menarche in girls when compared with siblings and population norms. Pubertal onset in boys was not affected, although boys were noted to have smaller testicular sizes and low/absent germ cells in testicular biopsies done at completion of therapy, despite receiving no gonadal radiation [20]. The finding that various pubertal milestones among girls may occur up to a year earlier than expected following 24 Gy cranial radiotherapy has since been confirmed by additional studies [21–24]. However, studies have not shown pubertal onset among boys to be significantly affected, although subtle differences in the magnitude or duration of the pubertal growth spurt may occur [22, 23].

Relatively few ALL patients currently receive cranial radiotherapy, and in those who do, a dose of 18 Gy now is preferentially used over 24 Gy [19]. Several studies have shown that this lower dose still is associated with earlier than expected attainment of pubertal milestones in girls [21, 25, 26], suggesting that if any safe threshold with regards to pubertal timing exists, it lies below 18 Gy. As with 24 Gy, onset of puberty in males does not appear to be significantly affected following 18 Gy cranial radiotherapy [27, 28]. A recent study from the large multi-institutional Childhood Cancer Survivor Study (CCSS) cohort showed that among almost 1,000 North American female ALL survivors, both <20 and ≥20 Gy cranial radiotherapy were associated with a 6-fold increased risk of subsequent early menarche (prior to age 10) compared with siblings [24]. In contrast, survivors treated with chemotherapy alone achieved menarche at a similar rate to siblings (fig. 1). Similar to findings among CNS tumor patients, younger age at exposure has also been associated with earlier onset of puberty among girls following 18 or 24 Gy radiotherapy for ALL.

Consequences of Early Puberty

Precocious puberty can lead to premature epiphyseal fusion, which causes shortening of the growth period and can result in adult short stature. The problem of short stature secondary to early puberty is exacerbated among patients exposed to cranial radiotherapy who have concurrent GH deficiency, especially after H-P doses ≥20 Gy [29, 30]. The evidence for GH deficiency following <20 Gy doses has been mixed [31, 32; see also Darzy and Shalet, pp 1–24]. Nevertheless, 18 Gy has been associated with a 4-fold increased risk of significant short adult stature (adult height >2 standard deviations below population average) compared with non-irradiated patients, albeit less than the almost 8-fold increased risk seen after higher doses of cranial radiotherapy [33]. Overall, females appear to be at greater risk of adult short stature compared with male survivors independent of radiotherapy dose (OR 3.0; 95% CI 2.2–4.2) [33]. These observations are consistent with survivors having decreased peak height velocities during their pubertal growth spurt [22, 23, 34].

Several unresolved issues remain. While most studies have focused on examining differences in the timing of specific pubertal milestones (e.g. menarche), the overall effect of treatment on total pubertal duration, or the tempo of puberty, remains less well studied. In longitudinal studies, the tempo of puberty was accelerated in some [20, 23, 25] but not all patient groups [22]. With an accelerated tempo, the duration of the pubertal growth spurt is shortened and there is less time to intervene medically to maximize final height. It is also unclear why girls are more susceptible to alterations in pubertal timing following radiotherapy compared with boys. Given that idiopathic precocious puberty also occurs more commonly in girls versus boys [35], some have postulated that female CNS control of pubertal timing may be more easily disrupted following any insult compared with

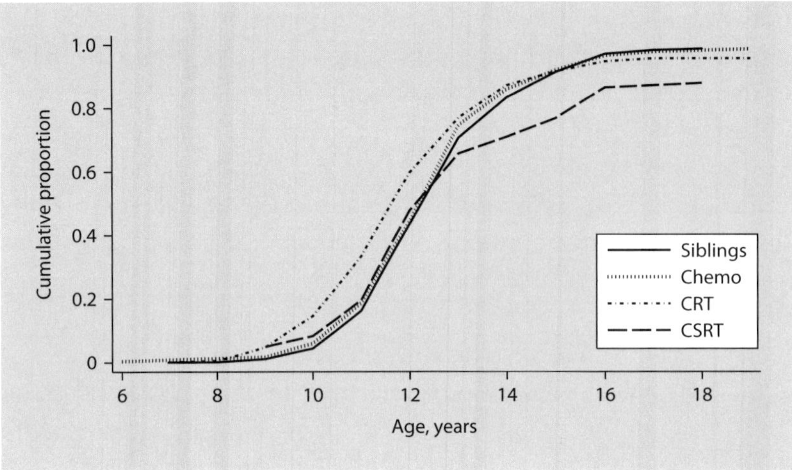

Fig. 1. Proportion of female survivors of childhood acute lymphoblastic leukemia who achieved menarche after diagnosis, adjusted for ethnicity, birth year, and abdominal radiotherapy [24]. Compared with siblings, survivors treated with chemotherapy only (Chemo) did not report menarche earlier (log rank test, $p = 0.76$), in contrast to those treated with cranial radiotherapy (CRT; $p < 0.01$). However, craniospinal radiotherapy (CSRT) was associated with delayed menarche compared with siblings ($p < 0.01$). Death and competing outcomes to menarche (e.g., hysterectomy) were not present in this cohort. Reproduced with permission from Chow et al. [24].

males. Nonetheless, the underlying physiologic mechanisms remain unknown [36, 37]. Precocious puberty in males following cancer therapy may also be underdiagnosed, as treatment-related damage to testes may result in smaller testicular size and a falsely reassuring physical examination [20].

Therefore, childhood cancer survivors, especially those who received any cranial radiotherapy at a young age, should be closely monitored for clinical signs of early pubertal development. In instances of a concerning physical examination, supporting laboratory data such as gonadotropin (FSH, LH) and sex hormone (estradiol in girls and testosterone in boys) levels, both basal and following stimulation with GnRH, can be obtained, along with a bone age. This is especially important in males since early physical changes (i.e. testicular enlargement) may not be apparent despite raised plasma concentrations of testosterone and an advancing bone age. Given that precocious puberty and GH deficiency frequently coexist, particularly following H-P radiation, GH testing should also be considered in any child demonstrating evidence of early onset of puberty. GnRH analogs have been used successfully to suppress precocious puberty in children, resulting in improved final heights [8]. In instances of precocious puberty and GH deficiency, early combination therapy with GnRH analogs and GH supplementation may offer the best chance towards achieving an individual's predicted genetic height potential [38].

Delayed Puberty

Gonadotropin Deficiency

Central Nervous System Tumors

Any tumor that arises in the H-P region places a patient at risk of multiple endocrinopathies, including precocious puberty (see above) but also hypogonadotropic hypogonadism, which can present as either delayed onset of puberty or as pubertal arrest. In a series of 36 patients with craniopharyngioma, 19% had delayed onset of puberty as a presenting symptom [11]. Other series have reported that even when puberty is normal in its timing, most patients have laboratory evidence of gonadotropin deficiency [39, 40]. Hypogonadotropic hypogonadism and delayed puberty can be a presenting symptom of other CNS tumors common to the suprasellar/hypothalamic region including: CNS germinoma, optic pathway gliomas (astrocytomas), and more rarely pituitary tumors and CNS involvement of Langerhans' cell histiocytosis [1].

Central Nervous System Radiation

CNS radiation remains a central therapeutic modality for children with tumors of the brain and spinal cord. As previously mentioned, whole brain radiation and/or focal radiation to the H-P axis place patients at risk not only for early puberty, but also for the gradual onset of H-P failure. Higher doses of radiation may cause gonadotropin deficiency and pubertal delay [41]. Radiation-induced hypopituitarism is dose-dependent. In an evaluation of 251 patients, there was a greater incidence of gonadotropin deficiency in patients who received 35–45 Gy compared to those who received only 20 Gy [42]. In a second study of 45 cases receiving CNS radiotherapy of up to 60 Gy, 14 patients either had delayed onset of puberty, lack of pubertal progression, or secondary amenorrhea [43].

Primary Ovarian and Leydig Cell Failure (Primary Deficiency of Sex Steroids)

Exposure of the ovary and testis to both radiotherapy and certain types of chemotherapy places children with cancer at an increased risk of primary gonadal failure. When exposure occurs in prepubertal children, the clinical manifestation may be delayed or absent puberty. Failure to enter or progress normally through puberty will ultimately result in other symptoms and problems including loss of libido and decreased bone mineral density in both sexes as well as erectile dysfunction, and decreased muscle mass in males [44].

Radiation-Induced Testicular Failure

Various studies suggest that the risk of Leydig cell failure is directly related to the dose of radiation delivered, with boys receiving 24–30 Gy at much higher risk than those receiving lower doses [44]. Additionally, several studies have demonstrated that younger age at the time of radiation is associated with an increased incidence of Leydig cell insufficiency [45–47].

The relative sparing of Leydig cell function in the setting of low and moderate doses of radiotherapy exposure was demonstrated by the Children's Cancer Study Group in an evaluation of 60 patients treated for childhood ALL [48]. Children received 18–24 Gy of radiation to one of three sites: craniospinal with an additional 12 Gy abdominal boost that included the gonads; craniospinal alone (no abdominal boost), or cranial radiotherapy. All groups received identical chemotherapy regimens. Only 1 patient had delayed pubertal development with low gonadotropin levels. Testosterone levels were generally unaffected, with 48 of 50 having normal levels for age. A number of smaller studies have corroborated these findings in the ALL population, however most additional studies are limited in size (8–15 patients) and do not control for the confounding effects of chemotherapy [49]. Studies that have evaluated the effects of radiation scatter in patients treated for Hodgkin's disease (17 patients, estimated testicular dose 0.2 Gy) and nephroblastoma (8 patients, estimated testicular dose 2–10 Gy) found few abnormalities in serum levels of LH or testosterone [50, 51].

A similar experience has been observed after bone marrow transplantations that have used total body irradiation (TBI) as part of the preparative therapy. Sarafoglou et al. [45] found that in a group of 17 boys treated with 13.7–15 Gy TBI with a 4-Gy testicular boost, only 1 patient experienced delayed onset of puberty with elevated levels of LH and FSH, and testosterone levels in the prepubertal range, consistent with Leydig cell failure. Notably, this patient was the only participant to receive a 12-Gy boost to the testis. In a second cohort of 41 males treated with TBI (10–12 Gy), Couto-Silva et al. [52] found that 3 patients demonstrated complete Leydig cell failure. Other evaluations of smaller populations found no cases of delayed puberty but occasional elevation of LH or low levels of testosterone [53, 54].

Young males who experience testicular relapse of ALL require higher doses of radiotherapy (24 Gy) to achieve reasonable cure rates and almost universally develop frank Leydig cell failure as a result. Brauner et al. [46] reported that only 2 of 21 patients with bilateral testicular radiation maintained normal Leydig cell function. Other investigators have reported that over 50% of such a population will experience pubertal delay with all patients having abnormally elevated levels of LH [55].

Radiation-Induced Ovarian Failure

Females treated with abdominal, pelvic, or spinal radiation are at significant risk of ovarian failure and the risk increases with increasing doses of radiation. The prroximity of the ovaries to the radiation field is an important risk factor. In a cohort of 182 female survivors of a heterogeneous group of childhood cancer diagnoses, 68% of patients who had both ovaries in the radiation field experienced ovarian failure. Only 14% of those whose ovaries were on the edge of the treatment field, and none of the patients whose ovaries were outside the radiation field experienced ovarian failure [56]. In an evaluation of 3,390 participants in the CCSS, doses of ovarian radiation of >10 Gy conferred a significant risk (OR 55; 95% CI 22.3–157.8) for acute ovarian failure defined as delayed/absent menarche or early termination of menses in the first 5 years after treatment [57]. Lower doses were associated with acute ovarian failure more commonly in the setting of exposure to cyclophosphamide or procarbazine. Unlike males, however, younger females are less likely than older females to experience ovarian failure at a given dose of ovarian radiation [57]. This is attributable to the fact that at birth there are approximately 1 million primordial follicles in the ovary, a number that drops to around 300,000 at the time puberty. This follicular reserve provides relative protection to the young, radiation-exposed female. Thus, the younger the patient the greater the dose needed to induce ovarian failure [44, 58]. However, the addition of alkylating agents may decrease the threshold dose of radiation required to induce ovarian failure.

Craniospinal radiation therapy used in females with ALL (18–24 Gy) may alter ovarian function. Hamre et al. [59] evaluated 97 female survivors of ALL and found that only those who got abdominal radiotherapy (12 Gy) in addition to craniospinal (18–24 Gy) were at risk of lack of pubertal development and late onset of menses. However, more recently, in a report from the CCSS of 949 female survivors of childhood ALL, craniospinal radiotherapy was associated with an increased risk of late onset menarche (OR 4.8; 95% CI 1.4–16.7; fig. 1) [24].

Females treated with abdominal or pelvic radiation, such as survivors of Wilms' tumor, Hodgkin's disease, or neuroblastoma, and female recipients of bone marrow transplantation often receive higher doses of ovarian radiation, often in combination with alkylating agents, and thus are at much greater risk of delayed or absent puberty. Doses of radiation to the whole abdomen of 20–30 Gy have resulted in 27 of 28 patients failing to undergo complete pubertal development [60]. In patients who have received oophoropexy or ovarian transposition, ovarian function may be preserved [61, 62]. However, almost 100% of patients who undergo TBI-based stem cell transplantation after age 10 will experience ovarian failure; young age is protective, however, such that only 50% of girls under 10 years of age are at risk [45, 63, 64].

Chemotherapy-Induced Leydig Cell Failure

The alkylating agents (including cyclophosphamide, ifosfamide, busulfan, cis-platinum, procarbazine, BCNU and CCNU), a class of chemotherapeutic agents that serve as the backbone of therapy for many common malignancies, are known to be gonadotoxic. It is clear, however, that the Leydig cell is not as sensitive as the germ cell to these gonadotoxic effects such that doses of alkylating agents that may induce sterility, are unlikely to affect testosterone production. In fact, early case series found normal testicular function and normal pubertal development after anti-leukemic therapy and only limited dysfunction in patients receiving bone marrow transplantation that included radiation exposure as well as alkylating chemotherapy [53, 65–67].

Traditionally, treatment of Hodgkin's disease has included alkylator-based drug combinations such as MOPP (includes mechlorethamine and procarbazine) and COPP (includes cyclophosphamide and procarbazine). Even so, studies of survivors of Hodgkin's disease receiving such therapy have not reported delayed onset of puberty among patients who have not received additional pelvic radiotherapy [68, 69]. In an evaluation of 209 male survivors of Hodgkin's disease treated with MVPP (mechlorethamine, vinblastine, procarbazine and prednisone) Howell et al. [70] reported normal mean testosterone values, but higher mean LH values (7.9 vs. 4.1, $p < 0.0001$) compared to controls. Fifty-two percent of participants had elevation of LH above the upper limit of normal suggesting that subclinical Leydig cell damage does occur. However, after the initial insult and LH elevation, a subsequent decline in LH values occurred in the 10 years following therapy, suggesting that some recovery of Leydig cell function does occur [70]. Memorial Sloan-Kettering reported a lower prevalence of both LH elevation (9%) and testosterone reduction (12%) after treatment with procarbazine and cyclophosphamide-based therapy (no mechlorethamine) [71, 72]. Overall, the risk of testicular dysfunction increases with increasing cumulative doses of alkylating agents, and when doses of known offending agents, such as mechlorethamine, are reduced, less gonadal damage is observed [73, 74]. Finally, alkylator-based therapy is commonly used in the treatment of other solid tumors, again, with minimal impact on pubertal timing [75]. Subclinical Leydig cell dysfunction has been noted after treatment of germ cell tumors with cis-platinum-based chemotherapy as well [76].

Chemotherapy-Induced Ovarian Failure

Similar to the late-effect profile of radiation therapy in females, and likewise, due to the relatively greater number of follicles in the ovary, young female patients treated with conventional chemotherapy are relatively more resistant than adolescents to ovarian failure manifested as either delayed or arrested puberty. In an evaluation of 35 survivors of childhood leukemia (peak incidence 2–5 years of age), 16 of the 17 girls who were prepubertal at the time of diagnosis had normal H-P-ovarian function, with a single patient experiencing pubertal arrest at Tanner stage 3 [77]. However, data from the multicenter CCSS study identified exposure to procarbazine at any age and exposure to cyclophosphamide at ages 13–20 as independent risk factors for ovarian failure among those treated for childhood cancer [57]. For individuals treated for tumors of the CNS, the addition of gonadotoxic agents such as procarbazine, CCNU, and BCNU to craniospinal radiation appears to increase the risk of ovarian failure and pubertal delay/arrest in this population [78].

Females who undergo myeloablative preparative therapy in the context of stem cell transplant that includes busulfan, thiotepa, or melphalan are also at high risk of ovarian failure and delayed/arrested puberty. Busulfan appears to be particularly toxic in that the majority of exposed females experience ovarian failure [79, 80]. Transplants performed with cyclophosphamide alone without busulfan are not associated with abnormalities in ovarian function [81].

Conclusion

Abnormalities of the timing of puberty are observed commonly in young children who are diagnosed and treated for cancer. Both early and delayed/arrested puberty can be seen. Precocious puberty occurs in association with certain tumors of the CNS and following H-P radiation. Delayed puberty may develop as a result of tumor- or radiation-induced LH/FSH deficiency or due to primary gonadal failure following exposure to alkylating agents and/or external beam radiation. These alterations of puberty can affect linear growth, skeletal health, and psychosexual development. As these disorders of puberty are amenable to a variety of medical interventions, it is essential that clinicians involved in the care of these children are aware of which children are at highest risk. Anticipatory surveillance of those at risk will enable early identification of problems and facilitate timely interventions, as clinically indicated.

Acknowledgements

Special thanks to Beverly Johnson and Dawn Silcott for the preparation of this manuscript. Financial support provided by the American Lebanese-Syrian Associated Charities (ALSAC).

References

1 Styne D, Grumbach MM: Puberty: ontogeny, neuroendocrinology, physiology, and disorders; in Kronenberg H (ed): Williams Textbook of Endocrinology, ed 11. Philadelphia, Saunders Elsevier, 2008, pp 969–1166.

2 Hewitt M, Weiner SL, Simone JV (eds): Childhood Cancer Survivorship: Improving Care and Quality of Life. Washington, National Academic Press, 2003.

3 Ries L, Eisner MP, Kosary CL: SEER Cancer Statistics Review, 1975–2002. Bethesda, National Cancer Institute, 2005.
4 Chumlea WC, Schubert CM, Roche AF, Kulin HE, Lee PA, Himes JH, Sun SS: Age at menarche and racial comparisons in US girls. Pediatrics 2003; 111:110–113.
5 Herman-Giddens ME, Kaplowitz PB, Wasserman R: Navigating the recent articles on girls' puberty in Pediatrics: what do we know and where do we go from here? Pediatrics 2004;113:911–917.
6 Whincup PH, Gilg JA, Odoki K, Taylor SJ, Cook DG: Age of menarche in contemporary British teenagers: survey of girls born between 1982 and 1986. BMJ 2001;322:1095–1096.
7 Tanner JM, Davies PS: Clinical longitudinal standards for height and height velocity for North American children. J Pediatr 1985;107:317–329.
8 Partsch CJ, Heger S, Sippell WG: Management and outcome of central precocious puberty. Clin Endocrinol (Oxf) 2002;56:129–148.
9 Bridges NA, Christopher JA, Hindmarsh PC, Brook CG: Sexual precocity: sex incidence and aetiology. Arch Dis Child 1994;70:116–118.
10 Trivin C, Couto-Silva AC, Sainte-Rose C, Chemaitilly W, Kalifa C, Doz F, Zerah M, Brauner R: Presentation and evolution of organic central precocious puberty according to the type of CNS lesion. Clin Endocrinol (Oxf) 2006;65:239–245.
11 de Vries L, Lazar L, Phillip M: Craniopharyngioma: presentation and endocrine sequelae in 36 children. J Pediatr Endocrinol Metab 2003;16: 703–710.
12 Garnett MR, Puget S, Grill J, Sainte-Rose C: Craniopharyngioma. Orphanet J Rare Dis 2007;2:18.
13 Sklar CA, Grumbach MM, Kaplan SL, Conte FA: Hormonal and metabolic abnormalities associated with central nervous system germinoma in children and adolescents and the effect of therapy: report of 10 patients. J Clin Endocrinol Metab 1981;52:9–16.
14 Ogilvy-Stuart AL, Clayton PE, Shalet SM: Cranial irradiation and early puberty. J Clin Endocrinol Metab 1994;78:1282–1286.
15 Oberfield SE, Soranno D, Nirenberg A, Heller G, Allen JC, David R, Levine LS, Sklar CA: Age at onset of puberty following high-dose central nervous system radiation therapy. Arch Pediatr Adolesc Med 1996;150:589–592.
16 Lannering B, Jansson C, Rosberg S, Albertsson-Wikland K: Increased LH and FSH secretion after cranial irradiation in boys. Med Pediatr Oncol 1997;29:280–287.
17 Constine LS, Woolf PD, Cann D, Mick G, McCormick K, Raubertas RF, Rubin P: Hypothalamic-pituitary dysfunction after radiation for brain tumors. N Engl J Med 1993;328:87–94.
18 Pai HH, Thornton A, Katznelson L, Finkelstein DM, Adams JA, Fullerton BC, Loeffler JS, Leibsch NJ, Klibanski A, Munzenrider JE: Hypothalamic/pituitary function following high-dose conformal radiotherapy to the base of skull: demonstration of a dose-effect relationship using dose-volume histogram analysis. Int J Radiat Oncol Biol Phys 2001;49:1079–1092.
19 Margolin JF, Steuber CP, Poplack DG: Acute lymphoblastic leukemia; in Pizzo PA, Poplack DG (eds): Principles and Practice of Pediatric Oncology. Philadelphia, Lippincott Williams & Wilkins, 2006, pp 538–590.
20 Quigley C, Cowell C, Jimenez M, Burger H, Kirk J, Bergin M, Stevens M, Simpson J, Silink M: Normal or early development of puberty despite gonadal damage in children treated for acute lymphoblastic leukemia. N Engl J Med 1989;321:143–151.
21 Moell C, Marky I, Hovi L, Kristinsson J, Rix M, Moe PJ, Garwicz S: Cerebral irradiation causes blunted pubertal growth in girls treated for acute leukemia. Med Pediatr Oncol 1994;22: 375–379.
22 Didcock E, Davies HA, Didi M, Ogilvy Stuart AL, Wales JK, Shalet SM: Pubertal growth in young adult survivors of childhood leukemia. J Clin Oncol 1995;13:2503–2507.
23 Groot-Loonen JJ, van Setten P, Otten BJ, van 't Hof MA, Lippens RJ, Stoelinga GB: Shortened and diminished pubertal growth in boys and girls treated for acute lymphoblastic leukaemia. Acta Paediatr 1996;85:1091–1095.
24 Chow EJ, Friedman DL, Yasui Y, Whitton JA, Stovall M, Robison LL, Sklar CA: Timing of menarche among survivors of childhood acute lymphoblastic leukemia: a report from the Childhood Cancer Survivor Study. Pediatr Blood Cancer 2008; 50:854–858.
25 Maneschi F, Fugardi MG, Corsello G, LoCurto M: Pubertal maturation in girls treated for childhood acute leukaemia. Eur J Pediatr 1991;150: 630–633.
26 Mills JL, Fears TR, Robison LL, Nicholson HS, Sklar CA, Byrne J: Menarche in a cohort of 188 long-term survivors of acute lymphoblastic leukemia. J Pediatr 1997;131:598–602.
27 Uruena M, Stanhope R, Chessells JM, Leiper AD: Impaired pubertal growth in acute lymphoblastic leukaemia. Arch Dis Child 1991;66:1403–1407.

28 Leiper AD, Stanhope R, Kitching P, Chessells JM: Precocious and premature puberty associated with treatment of acute lymphoblastic leukaemia. Arch Dis Child 1987;62:1107–1112.
29 Stubberfield TG, Byrne GC, Jones TW: Growth and growth hormone secretion after treatment for acute lymphoblastic leukemia in childhood. 18-Gy versus 24-Gy cranial irradiation. J Pediatr Hematol Oncol 1995;17:167–171.
30 Birkebaek NH, Fisker S, Clausen N, Tuovinen V, Sindet-Pedersen S, Christiansen JS: Growth and endocrinological disorders up to 21 years after treatment for acute lymphoblastic leukemia in childhood. Med Pediatr Oncol 1998;30:351–356.
31 Melin AE, Adan L, Leverger G, Souberbielle JC, Schaison G, Brauner R: Growth hormone secretion, puberty and adult height after cranial irradiation with 18 Gy for leukaemia. Eur J Pediatr 1998;157:703–707.
32 Hata M, Ogino I, Aida N, Saito K, Omura M, Kigasawa H, Toyoda Y, Tachibana K, Matsubara S, Inoue T: Prophylactic cranial irradiation of acute lymphoblastic leukemia in childhood: outcomes of late effects on pituitary function and growth in long-term survivors. Int J Cancer 2001;96(suppl): 117–124.
33 Chow EJ, Friedman DL, Yasui Y, Whitton JA, Stovall M, Robison LL, Sklar CA: Decreased adult height in survivors of childhood acute lymphoblastic leukemia: a report from the Childhood Cancer Survivor Study. J Pediatr 2007;150:370–375, 375.e371.
34 Hokken-Koelega AC, van Doorn JW, Hahlen K, Stijnen T, de Muinck Keizer-Schrama SM, Drop SL: Long-term effects of treatment for acute lymphoblastic leukemia with and without cranial irradiation on growth and puberty: a comparative study. Pediatr Res 1993;33:577–582.
35 Kaplowitz P: Precocious puberty: update on secular trends, definitions, diagnosis, and treatment. Adv Pediatr 2004;51:37–62.
36 Darzy KH, Shalet SM: Hypopituitarism as a consequence of brain tumours and radiotherapy. Pituitary 2005;8:203–211.
37 Armstrong GT, Sklar CA, Hudson MM, Robison LL: Long-term health status among survivors of childhood cancer: does sex matter? J Clin Oncol 2007;25:4477–4489.
38 Gleeson HK, Stoeter R, Ogilvy-Stuart AL, Gattamaneni HR, Brennan BM, Shalet SM: Improvements in final height over 25 years in growth hormone (GH)-deficient childhood survivors of brain tumors receiving GH replacement. J Clin Endocrinol Metab 2003;88:3682–3689.
39 Rivarola MA, Mendilaharzu H, Warman M, Belgorosky A, Iorcansky S, Castellano M, Caresana A, Chaler E, Maceiras M: Endocrine disorders in 66 suprasellar and pineal tumors of patients with prepubertal and pubertal ages. Horm Res 1992;37:1–6.
40 Sanford RA, Muhlbauer MS: Craniopharyngioma in children. Neurol Clin 1991;9:453–465.
41 Toogood AA: Endocrine consequences of brain irradiation. Growth Horm IGF Res 2004;14(suppl A):S118–S124.
42 Littley MD, Shalet SM, Beardwell CG, Robinson EL, Sutton ML: Radiation-induced hypopituitarism is dose-dependent. Clin Endocrinol (Oxf) 1989;31:363–373.
43 Rappaport R, Brauner R, Czernichow P, Thibaud E, Renier D, Zucker JM, Lemerle J: Effect of hypothalamic and pituitary irradiation on pubertal development in children with cranial tumors. J Clin Endocrinol Metab 1982;54:1164–1168.
44 Sklar C: Reproductive physiology and treatment-related loss of sex hormone production. Med Pediatr Oncol 1999;33:2–8.
45 Sarafoglou K, Boulad F, Gillio A, Sklar C: Gonadal function after bone marrow transplantation for acute leukemia during childhood. J Pediatr 1997;130:210–216.
46 Brauner R, Caltabiano P, Rappaport R, Leverger G, Schaison G: Leydig cell insufficiency after testicular irradiation for acute lymphoblastic leukemia. Horm Res 1988;30:111–114.
47 Shalet SM, Tsatsoulis A, Whitehead E, Read G: Vulnerability of the human Leydig cell to radiation damage is dependent upon age. J Endocrinol 1989;120:161–165.
48 Sklar CA, Robison LL, Nesbit ME, Sather HN, Meadows AT, Ortega JA, Kim TH, Hammond GD: Effects of radiation on testicular function in long-term survivors of childhood acute lymphoblastic leukemia: a report from the Children Cancer Study Group. J Clin Oncol 1990;8:1981–1987.
49 Castillo LA, Craft AW, Kernahan J, Evans RG, Aynsley-Green A: Gonadal function after 12-Gy testicular irradiation in childhood acute lymphoblastic leukaemia. Med Pediatr Oncol 1990;18: 185–189.
50 Shalet SM, Beardwell CG, Jacobs HS, Pearson D: Testicular function following irradiation of the human prepubertal testis. Clin Endocrinol (Oxf) 1978;9:483–490.

51 Kinsella TJ, Trivette G, Rowland J, Sorace R, Miller R, Fraass B, Steinberg SM, Glatstein E, Sherins RJ: Long-term follow-up of testicular function following radiation therapy for early-stage Hodgkin's disease. J Clin Oncol 1989;7:718–724.

52 Couto-Silva AC, Trivin C, Thibaud E, Esperou H, Michon J, Brauner R: Factors affecting gonadal function after bone marrow transplantation during childhood. Bone Marrow Transplant 2001;28: 67–75.

53 Sklar CA, Kim TH, Ramsay NK: Testicular function following bone marrow transplantation performed during or after puberty. Cancer 1984;53: 1498–1501.

54 Bakker B, Massa GG, Oostdijk W, Van Weel-Sipman MH, Vossen JM, Wit JM: Pubertal development and growth after total-body irradiation and bone marrow transplantation for haematological malignancies. Eur J Pediatr 2000;159:31–37.

55 Leiper AD, Grant DB, Chessells JM: Gonadal function after testicular radiation for acute lymphoblastic leukaemia. Arch Dis Child 1986;61:53–56.

56 Stillman RJ, Schinfeld JS, Schiff I, Gelber RD, Greenberger J, Larson M, Jaffe N, Li FP: Ovarian failure in long-term survivors of childhood malignancy. Am J Obstet Gynecol 1981;139:62–66.

57 Chemaitilly W, Mertens AC, Mitby P, Whitton J, Stovall M, Yasui Y, Robison LL, Sklar CA: Acute ovarian failure in the childhood cancer survivor study. J Clin Endocrinol Metab 2006;91:1723–1728.

58 Wallace WH, Thomson AB, Saran F, Kelsey TW: Predicting age of ovarian failure after radiation to a field that includes the ovaries. Int J Radiat Oncol Biol Phys 2005;62:738–744.

59 Hamre MR, Robison LL, Nesbit ME, Sather HN, Meadows AT, Ortega JA, D'Angio GJ, Hammond GD: Effects of radiation on ovarian function in long-term survivors of childhood acute lymphoblastic leukemia: a report from the Children's Cancer Study Group. J Clin Oncol 1987;5:1759–1765.

60 Wallace WH, Shalet SM, Crowne EC, Morris-Jones PH, Gattamaneni HR: Ovarian failure following abdominal irradiation in childhood: natural history and prognosis. Clin Oncol (R Coll Radiol) 1989;1:75–79.

61 Ortin TT, Shostak CA, Donaldson SS: Gonadal status and reproductive function following treatment for Hodgkin's disease in childhood: the Stanford experience. Int J Radiat Oncol Biol Phys 1990;19:873–880.

62 Thibaud E, Ramirez M, Brauner R, Flamant F, Zucker JM, Fekete C, Rappaport R: Preservation of ovarian function by ovarian transposition performed before pelvic irradiation during childhood. J Pediatr 1992;121:880–884.

63 Sklar C: Growth and endocrine disturbances after bone marrow transplantation in childhood. Acta Paediatr Suppl 1995;411:57–62.

64 Sanders JE, Buckner CD, Amos D, Levy W, Appelbaum FR, Doney K, Storb R, Sullivan KM, Witherspoon RP, Thomas ED: Ovarian function following marrow transplantation for aplastic anemia or leukemia. J Clin Oncol 1988;6:813–818.

65 Blatt J, Poplack DG, Sherins RJ: Testicular function in boys after chemotherapy for acute lymphoblastic leukemia. N Engl J Med 1981;304: 1121–1124.

66 Sklar CA: Growth and pubertal development in survivors of childhood cancer. Pediatrician 1991; 18:53–60.

67 Shalet SM, Hann IM, Lendon M, Morris Jones PH, Beardwell CG: Testicular function after combination chemotherapy in childhood for acute lymphoblastic leukaemia. Arch Dis Child 1981, 56:275–278.

68 Mackie EJ, Radford M, Shalet SM. Gonadal function following chemotherapy for childhood Hodgkin's disease. Med Pediatr Oncol 1996;27: 74–78.

69 Kulkarni SS, Sastry PS, Saikia TK, Parikh PM, Gopal R, Advani SH: Gonadal function following ABVD therapy for Hodgkin's disease. Am J Clin Oncol 1997;20:354–357.

70 Howell SJ, Radford JA, Ryder WD, Shalet SM: Testicular function after cytotoxic chemotherapy: evidence of Leydig cell insufficiency. J Clin Oncol 1999;17:1493–1498.

71 Papadakis V, Vlachopapadopoulou E, Van Syckle K, Ganshaw L, Kalmanti M, Tan C, Sklar C: Gonadal function in young patients successfully treated for Hodgkin disease. Med Pediatr Oncol 1999;32:366–372.

72 Greenfield DM, Walters SJ, Coleman RE, Hancock BW, Eastell R, Davies HA, Snowden JA, Derogatis L, Shalet SM, Ross RJ: Prevalence and consequences of androgen deficiency in young male cancer survivors in a controlled cross-sectional study. J Clin Endocrinol Metab 2007;92: 3476–3482.

73 van den Berg H, Furstner F, van den Bos C, Behrendt H: Decreasing the number of MOPP courses reduces gonadal damage in survivors of childhood Hodgkin disease. Pediatr Blood Cancer 2004;42:210–215.

74 Bramswig JH, Heimes U, Heiermann E, Schlegel W, Nieschlag E, Schellong G: The effects of different cumulative doses of chemotherapy on testicular function. Results in 75 patients treated for Hodgkin's disease during childhood or adolescence. Cancer 1990;65:1298–1302.
75 Aubier F, Flamant F, Brauner R, Caillaud JM, Chaussain JM, Lemerle J: Male gonadal function after chemotherapy for solid tumors in childhood. J Clin Oncol 1989;7:304–309.
76 Brennemann W, Stoffel-Wagner B, Helmers A, Mezger J, Jager N, Klingmuller D: Gonadal function of patients treated with cisplatin based chemotherapy for germ cell cancer. J Urol 1997;158:844–850.
77 Siris ES, Leventhal BG, Vaitukaitis JL: Effects of childhood leukemia and chemotherapy on puberty and reproductive function in girls. N Engl J Med 1976;294:1143–1146.
78 Clayton PE, Shalet SM, Price DA, Jones PH: Ovarian function following chemotherapy for childhood brain tumours. Med Pediatr Oncol 1989;17:92–96.
79 Thibaud E, Rodriguez-Macias K, Trivin C, Esperou H, Michon J, Brauner R: Ovarian function after bone marrow transplantation during childhood. Bone Marrow Transplant 1998;21:287–290.
80 Teinturier C, Hartmann O, Valteau-Couanet D, Benhamou E, Bougneres PF: Ovarian function after autologous bone marrow transplantation in childhood: high-dose busulfan is a major cause of ovarian failure. Bone Marrow Transplant 1998;22:989–994.
81 Sanders JE, Hawley J, Levy W, Gooley T, Buckner CD, Deeg HJ, Doney K, Storb R, Sullivan K, Witherspoon R, Appelbaum FR: Pregnancies following high-dose cyclophosphamide with or without high-dose busulfan or total-body irradiation and bone marrow transplantation. Blood 1996;87:3045–3052.

Gregory T. Armstrong, MD
Department of Epidemiology and Cancer Control, St. Jude Children's Research Hospital
332 North Lauderdale Street, Mail Stop 735
Memphis, TN 38105 (USA)
Tel. +1 901 495 5892, Fax +1 901 495 5845, E-Mail greg.armstrong@stjude.org

Wallace WHB, Kelnar CJH (eds): Endocrinopathy after Childhood Cancer Treatment.
Endocr Dev. Basel, Karger, 2009, vol 15, pp 40–58

Obesity during and after Treatment for Childhood Cancer

John J. Reilly

Division of Developmental Medicine, Yorkhill Hospitals, University of Glasgow, Glasgow, UK

Abstract

Obesity is a common complication of treatment for some childhood cancers, particularly acute lymphoblastic leukaemia (ALL) and craniopharyngioma. Evidence-based guidance is available for the general paediatric population on the diagnosis, aetiology, consequences, prevention and treatment of obesity, and this should be considered as the starting point for considering such issues in patients with malignancy. In ALL, a high proportion of patients show rapid and excessive weight gain soon after diagnosis which originates partly in lifestyle, in particular via markedly reduced levels of physical activity. Good evidence on risk factors for obesity in ALL is available, and the natural history and aetiology of obesity in ALL are now fairly well understood, while for craniopharyngioma the natural history is reasonably well understood. Understanding the natural history and aetiology of obesity should facilitate preventive interventions in the future. Evidence on preventive interventions is required urgently, and it should focus on promotion of a reduction in sedentary behaviour and increases in physical activity. Such interventions should be helpful in obesity prevention, but could also have a wide range of additional benefits in the prevention or amelioration of other late effects of treatment.

An epidemic of paediatric obesity has occurred across the developed world and much of the developing world in recent years [1]. There are subgroups within the population at high-risk of becoming obese, notably patients treated for some childhood cancers [1]. Children treated for childhood cancer may also be at unusually high risk from the consequences of obesity, particularly the cardiovascular and metabolic comorbidities. In addition, there is emerging evidence that obesity might be an adverse prognostic factor in some childhood malignancies.

The present review is a summary and critique of recent reviews of obesity in the general paediatric population, and obesity in childhood cancer, which aims to:

(1) Summarise recent systematic reviews on the diagnosis, aetiology, consequences, prevention and treatment of obesity in the general population

(2) Summarise recent evidence on the development of obesity during and after childhood cancer
(3) Critically appraise the evidence on obesity during and after childhood cancer, identifying major gaps in the literature, and identifying opportunities which have been provided by recent improvements in study design and methodology

Obesity in the General Paediatric Population

Recent systematic reviews have produced evidence-based guidance on most aspects of childhood obesity [2–5], and expert committee recommendations are also available [6–8]. In this section brief and critical reviews of this material are provided.

Diagnosis and Definitions of Paediatric Obesity

Obesity is a body fat content which is sufficiently high as to increase risk of disease. This definition has two components: body fat content, and risk of disease or 'comorbidity'. In routine clinical practice and many research settings, direct measurement of body fat content is impractical and so there is a need for simpler proxy indices of fatness. There are currently two candidate proxy measures: the body mass index (BMI), and waist circumference. These two measures in turn have several variants. In paediatric applications the BMI usually has to be expressed as a percentile or standard deviation (SD) score (z score) relative to population reference data since BMI changes markedly with age, and differs between the sexes. Systematic reviews of the diagnostic evidence on childhood obesity have concluded that a high BMI for age (such as BMI ≥95th percentile) is a good diagnostic marker for both a high fat mass and risk of comorbid conditions [9]. Children defined as obese in this way, with a high BMI for age and sex, are almost always excessively fat, i.e., this definition has high diagnostic specificity (low false-positive rate). The high specificity makes the definition particularly appropriate for clinical use [7], since it is important to avoid diagnosing obesity in the non-obese child or adolescent. Systematic reviews have concluded that the *sensitivity* of a high BMI for age as a diagnostic criterion or definition is somewhat lower, giving a moderate to high false-negative rate which is dependent on the precise percentile cut-off chosen to define obesity [9]. The moderate sensitivity means that a relatively high proportion of excessively fat children will not have high BMIs for their age and sex and BMI-based definitions of paediatric obesity tend to be conservative [9, 10]: the true prevalence of excess fatness will usually be underestimated when obesity is defined using the BMI, and this appears to be true for the general paediatric population as well as children with diseases including those with childhood cancer [10].

The principal alternative to using national population reference data and percentiles of BMI involves an 'international' definition of obesity based on BMI. The international definition [11] aims to provide an age- and sex-specific value of BMI which is conceptually equivalent to adult definitions of obesity based on BMI (BMI of 30.0 at age 18 years). Systematic review has shown that using the international definition of obesity is highly conservative because sensitivity is even lower than when using national (percentile) definitions of obesity based on BMI [9], and estimates of prevalence of obesity when using the international definitions are usually much lower than when using national/BMI percentile definitions of obesity. A further problem when using the international definitions of obesity is that all four studies which have compared the diagnostic accuracy of national versus international definitions of obesity based on BMI have found that the sensitivity of the international obesity definition differs significantly between boys and girls, so that it does not provide an obesity definition which is equivalent between the sexes [9]. In the UK for example, the international definition has much lower sensitivity for the diagnosis of high fatness in boys than in girls and it produces artefactual differences in obesity prevalence between the sexes. For these reasons, and a variety of others [12], the international definition of obesity is not suitable for clinical use and has a number of disadvantages for research use including the low apparent prevalence of obesity and reduced power in applications which depend on the number of children or adolescents defined as obese, such as studies of the aetiology of obesity. However, international comparisons of obesity prevalence in childhood cancer might be facilitated by use of a standard international definition, and some journals now require that the international definition of obesity is used when reporting prevalence of obesity.

In adults, the traditional definition of obesity, based on BMI, has been superseded by definitions based on waist circumference, largely because of the evidence that waist circumference measures provide greater predictive validity for the cardiovascular and metabolic comorbidities of obesity [13]. This emergence of waist as the best simple proxy measure of obesity in adults has led to increased interest in the use of waist circumference as a means of defining or diagnosing obesity in children and adolescents, in part because of the implicit assumption that, as in adults, waist measurements would provide improved diagnostic accuracy/predictive validity for high fat mass or the cardiovascular comorbidities of obesity, or both. Recent systematic reviews and expert committee recommendations on the diagnosis of obesity in children and adolescents have noted that there is a lack of empirical paediatric evidence on the diagnostic accuracy of waist circumference [2, 3, 7, 8] and so the extent to which diagnosis might be improved by adding a measure of waist to BMI, or by replacing BMI with waist measurement, is unclear. The evidence-based guides and expert committee recommendations have consistently avoided recommending waist as a definition of obesity because of this lack of empirical evidence. However, three very recent paediatric studies which have made direct comparisons of the ability of BMI versus waist to diagnose high fat mass or cardiovascular risk factors have all found no improvements in accuracy when using waist [14–16] and early indications are that waist circumference measurement will not provide the benefits for diagnosis of paediatric obesity which have been demonstrated in adult obesity.

In summary, a high BMI for age and sex provides a practical and evidence-based means of defining childhood obesity which has high diagnostic accuracy.

Aetiology of Obesity in the General Paediatric Population

Obesity can only arise from a chronic state of positive energy balance, an excess of energy (food) intake over total energy expenditure, a reduction of total energy expenditure, or both. In growing children and adolescents a very small daily energy imbalance is required for normal growth (the energy cost of deposition of new tissue) and so an excess positive energy balance is that which is in addition to the requirement for growth. When considered in terms of energy imbalance in this way, the aetiology of obesity appears very simple. In fact, the aetiology of obesity in the general paediatric population is complex and the principal causes of the paediatric obesity epidemic remain poorly understood for a variety of reasons which are beyond the scope of the current review but discussed elsewhere [17]. In the general paediatric population only a few behaviours are well established as being causally involved in the obesity epidemic, and even these are contested. The behaviours which are well-established causes of obesity are: formula-feeding in infancy; rapid growth in infancy and early childhood; high consumption of sugar-sweetened drinks; high levels of sedentary behaviour (such as TV viewing and other forms of screen-time or media use) [18]. In addition, more recent evidence suggests that both reduced sleep duration and low levels of physical activity are also causally involved in the development of obesity [17].

If modifiable, these behaviours should form the basis of strategies for obesity prevention in children and adolescents, at least until our understanding of the aetiology of paediatric obesity improves [17]. For patients during and after treatment of childhood cancer a good deal of specific evidence on aetiology and natural history is available, particularly in acute lymphoblastic leukaemia (ALL). This evidence should inform strategies for prevention of obesity and reductions in cardiovascular risk and this evidence is summarised below, together with a discussion of gaps in this evidence and methodological improvements which might address these gaps.

Consequences of Paediatric Obesity in the General Population

A systematic review published in 2003, which reviewed evidence published up to the end of 2001, concluded that paediatric obesity had a wide variety of adverse consequences both in the short-term (for the obese child or adolescent) and the longer-term (for the adult who was obese as a child or adolescent) [4]. More recent evidence on the short-term effects of childhood obesity has been accumulating and is alarming. The most recent evidence has concerned the emergence of relatively common comorbidities which were thought previously to be rare, or comorbidities which were unknown previously. The evidence of a surprisingly high prevalence of fatty liver [19] and of widespread impairments in health-related quality of life [17, 18] is of particular concern, together with accumulating evidence of other adverse psychosocial effects particularly common in girls.

Evidence on the long-term impact of child or adolescent obesity on adult mortality remains scarce, largely because long-term follow-up of cohorts from childhood or adolescence to obesity has been scarce and such cohorts are usually small. In addition, some of the evidence on the effects of paediatric obesity on adult morbidity and premature mortality is apparently contradictory [22, 23], and there is a need for further research in this area, with greater emphasis on adjustment of associations between paediatric obesity and adult outcomes for adult weight status [24]. However, there is a large body of high quality evidence that obesity which is established early is persistent, and only a minority of obese adolescents in contemporary Western societies are likely to 'grow out of' their obesity [25, 26] and this is a particular concern for patients treated for some childhood cancers where the development of obesity occurs both commonly and rapidly by adolescence.

In summary, the health, social, and economic impact of paediatric obesity is substantial. The principal adverse consequences of paediatric obesity are summarised in table 1.

Evidence on Prevention and Treatment of Paediatric Obesity in the General Population

Systematic reviews of the evidence on specific interventions for the prevention and/or treatment of paediatric obesity have been critical [2, 3, 27, 28], concluding that evidence on specific interventions has been generally of poor quality, short-term (leaving doubts about the sustainability of interventions and their effects), and focused on testing interventions which often lack generalisability to other settings. Despite these concerns over weaknesses in the published evidence, improved evidence is likely to be available soon, given the plethora of preventive and treatment intervention studies now underway. In the meantime some 'best-bets' in obesity prevention and treatment are available, endorsed by expert committees and in evidence-based guidance [2, 5, 6–8]. Summaries of the 'best-bets' in obesity prevention and treatment are given in table 2.

One emerging observation in paediatric obesity treatment is that effects of treatment on BMI and bodyweight which can be achieved by traditional, fairly low intensity treatments are probably modest, in the order of <0.3 units in BMI SD

Table 1. Principal consequences of childhood obesity

Short term (for the obese child or adolescent)
Presence and clustering of cardiovascular risk factors
Low health-related quality of life
Increased risk of several orthopaedic abnormalities
Increased risk of diabetes
Increased risk of fatty liver
Lower self-esteem, particularly in girls
Long term (for the adult obese as a child or adolescent)
Persistence of obesity
Continuation or amplification of cardiovascular risk factors
Socio-economic and educational disadvantage, particularly in women
(Possible) premature mortality

score/6–12 months [29–31]. While most evidence-based treatment guides recommend weight maintenance as a goal of treatment, the empirical evidence suggests that weight maintenance is uncommon [29–31]. This relatively modest effect of most treatment programmes on weight status in obese children and adolescents implies that treatments should be offered over more prolonged periods, perhaps a year or more. Alternatively, more intense treatments might be indicated if more marked effects on weight status have to be achieved, or treatments might have to commence much earlier to achieve greater impact on weight status measures, when patients are younger and before obesity has become well established [31].

The effect size of treatment which is desirable is currently unknown and needs further study, but a reduction of >0.5 SD score units in BMI per year has been proposed as a possible target as it has been associated with statistically significant reductions in cardiovascular risk factors in a single study [33]. Most office-based treatments in the UK have been unable to achieve such sizeable effects on BMI, and more intensive treatments are likely to be required to achieve such effects more consistently, though the intensity of such treatments will compromise their generalisability [29].

As examples of the two extreme ends of the treatment spectrum from recent paediatric obesity treatment randomised controlled trials are the Scottish Childhood Overweight Treatment Programme ('SCOTT') which offered patients around 6 h of office-based treatment over 6 months [29] and achieved reductions in BMI SD score of around 0.2 units over 1 year, while the much more intensive 'Bright-Bodies' [32] treatment programme in the USA invested >70 h of treatment over the same period which might explain their greater treatment effects on BMI at 6 and 12 months.

Table 2. Evidence-based best bets in childhood obesity treatment and prevention

	Treatment	Prevention
Promote reduction in sedentary behaviour, to <2 h/day	Important	Important
Dietary modification	Essential	Desirable, not essential
Promotion of physical activity	Desirable	Desirable
Family self-monitoring of lifestyle	Desirable	Desirable

Despite this indication that effects of office-based obesity treatment might be modest, two aspects of recent evidence from paediatric obesity treatment randomised controlled trials are encouraging. First, the evidence that treatment has not had adverse effects: the perception that treatment might be harmful is a widespread barrier to treatment. Second, in most trials the psychosocial comorbidities of obesity, such as impaired quality of life, have *improved* with treatment. These psychosocial improvements may be of particular importance to families and patients because it is generally the psychosocial comorbidities which most concern patients and families [34, 35] rather than the cardiovascular and metabolic risk factors which are usually of greatest concern to health professionals.

In summary, modest benefits in the treatment of paediatric obesity are likely for weight-based measures and more marked improvements in other outcomes might be achieved even in relatively low intensity office-based treatments. More intense treatments, which last for prolonged periods, are likely to have greater impact on weight status. The generalisability of these findings, from treatment of the general paediatric population to treatment of obesity in children or adolescents during or after treatment for childhood cancer, is unclear as a result of lack of evidence from intervention studies in this group.

Obesity during and after Treatment for Childhood Cancer

Prevalence and Risk of Obesity during and after Treatment for Childhood Cancer
Reviews of the prevalence of obesity in childhood cancer have concluded consistently that the evidence is complex [36–38], and this is not surprising given the heterogeneity of diseases, treatments and outcomes, small sample sizes, and wide variations in definitions of obesity used and rapid secular trends to increased obesity prevalence in the general paediatric population. However, in ALL, the childhood malignancy which has received most attention in terms of obesity research, the evidence for disturbances of energy balance and obesity is substantial [36–39].

Even on recent treatment protocols, which avoid cranial radiotherapy (CRT) for the majority of patients, the prevalence obesity in ALL increased markedly by 5- to 10-fold during treatment [38] to levels much higher than the general paediatric population in most studies. With the high and increasing prevalence of paediatric obesity, even if the prevalence was the same in patients with childhood cancer as in the general population, this would be a major cause for concern, particularly given the cardiovascular, metabolic, musculoskeletal, psychosocial, and other sequelae which survivors of childhood cancer face [40] and which obesity would contribute to or exacerbate. In addition, if obesity affects prognosis of childhood cancer treatment (discussed below), obesity prevention and treatment will assume greater significance in childhood cancer treatment.

Other paediatric groups being treated for cancer are known to be at increased risk of obesity, notably those with tumours in the hypothalamo-pituitary region [38]. For patients treated for other malignancies the risk of early or late obesity is less well established, and in at least some groups, there is an unusually high prevalence of underweight in long-term survivors [37]. Much more research is required on the prevalence of underweight, overweight, and obesity during and after childhood cancer treatment, and comments aimed at informing such research are provided below.

A few methodological issues are worth noting when attempting to interpret data on the prevalence of underweight, overweight, and obesity in children being treated for cancer, or the long-term survivors of childhood cancer. First, as noted above, a high BMI for age is an accurate and evidence-based means of identifying obesity in children, adolescents, and young adults. In older adult survivors a BMI of ≥30.0 or an abnormally high waist circumference [13] provide simple but acceptable definitions of obesity. Since obesity prevalence is generally high and increasing rapidly [1], the prevalence of obesity in any patient group should be compared against age- and sex-matched prevalence estimates from the general population (ideally these would be available from national surveys or other forms of obesity surveillance) at around the same time in order to test for any excess of obesity in the patient population. Second, sample size considerations will affect the confidence of estimates of prevalence markedly [41]: generally samples of around 300–500 per age/sex group are required for precise estimates of obesity prevalence, though this depends on the prevalence, and similarly large samples are required to identify trends in obesity with confidence [42]. Most sample sizes in the paediatric cancer literature have been far smaller than this, and future research should place greater emphasis on using multicentre and/or national cohorts of treatment trial data [43] when generating estimates of obesity prevalence in order to increase confidence in estimates of prevalence and trends in prevalence. Studies using data which are collected routinely in childhood cancer treatment (weight and height, to permit calculation of BMI) can be extremely valuable in establishing a prevalence of obesity, changes in prevalence during and after treatment, and can also provide valuable insights into natural history and aetiology (discussed below).

If no national surveillance data are available to provide estimates of obesity prevalence in the general population at around the same time, a healthy control group will be required. Since the prevalence of obesity in some societies varies markedly by age, gender, ethnic group, and socioeconomic status [41], all these issues should be considered when a sample is being selected to provide a healthy control group.

Using data from the entire population of patients on a particular trial protocol should provide a relatively large sample size, and the estimates of prevalence generated from cohorts of patients can be provided for specified time periods (important given secular trends to a rapidly increasing prevalence of obesity [1]), and for specified treatment regimes – for example, protocols with vs. without use of CRT – important given the likely contribution of treatment regimens to obesity risk.

The use of more sophisticated and direct measures of body composition (rather than dependence on proxies for body composition such as BMI) can provide insights into the prevalence and aetiology of obesity not available when BMI is used [17, 36, 44–46]. However, since methods such as dual energy X-ray absorptiometry (DEXA) are more sophisticated and less practical than the simple proxy measures, their use inevitably tends to reduce sample size and will usually compromise study power. Use of body composition measures is probably best seen as being complementary to surveys of obesity prevalence based on BMI relative to national BMI reference data [9, 14], though the availability of DEXA, and its application for assessment of bone health, make it an appealing and useful option.

Aetiology and Natural History of Obesity during and after Treatment for Childhood Cancer

Most of the evidence on the aetiology and natural history of obesity in childhood cancer has come from studies of patients with ALL. This section will therefore focus on ALL, though much of this evidence has relevance to patients with other malignancies, and some specific evidence from studies of patients with other malignancies will be discussed, particularly from studies of patients with hypothalamo-pituitary tumours.

Understanding of the aetiology of obesity should, ideally begin with an understanding of its natural history: the timing of onset; rate of development, and the relationship to other events (such as cancer treatments) [17, 37]. In patients with ALL treated on European treatment protocols in the 1980s and 1990s the natural history of obesity is well described and has been reviewed elsewhere [38]. The 'natural history' studies have shown that patient groups with ALL proceed from normal weight status or mild underweight at diagnosis to overweight or obesity by the end of treatment. The prevalence of obesity increases 5- to 10-fold *during* treatment for ALL regardless of whether CRT was used, so that obesity prevalence is extremely high at the end of treatment and most patients, including those who do not become obese, show substantial and rapid excess weight gain *during* treatment [37, 38]. Descriptions of the natural history of obesity of this kind inform aetiological studies in many ways, by permitting the identification and study of patients, and in the 'pre-obese' state for example [47], which is an important paradigm in understanding aetiology of obesity. Good understanding of natural history also permits tests for causes of energy imbalance which might be specific to certain treatments or treatment periods, such as corticosteroid-induced increases in energy intake at specific times [48].

In summary, the evidence from patients with ALL indicates that most patients, regardless of CRT treatment, undergo a substantial positive energy balance during the course of treatment, and in most studies patients have tended to maintain their excess weight gain, or even continue to gain excess weight, after the end of treatment [38]. The origins of obesity in ALL, widely seen as a 'late-effect' of treatment, actually occur early. This is in keeping with contemporary studies on the aetiology of obesity in the general paediatric population where early origins of obesity are well established [17, 49]. Obesity often has early origins for a variety of reasons: the early adoption and establishment of 'obesogenic' behaviours, and early events which might 'programme' the regulation of long-term energy balance in an unfavourable direction.

Natural history studies in patients with childhood craniopharyngioma have also been extremely valuable in elucidating the timing and causes of obesity development in relation to treatment events such as surgery [50, 51]. The numbers of patients available for natural history studies of the development of obesity in rare malignancies will inevitably be small, but in many patient groups the natural history (for example the trajectory of BMI SD changes) is likely to be both striking and consistent, and patterns may be discernible even by studying relatively small numbers of patients longitudinally with simple indices such as BMI [38, 50, 51]. Where access to larger numbers are available – whole national or international cohorts of patients treated on the same or similar protocols for example – study of the natural history of obesity development will be even more informative. Repeated natural history studies of this kind are likely to be required over time as treatment protocols change and the as the wider environment continues to become more 'obesogenic' [1].

Development of Obesity in Patients during and after Treatment for Childhood Cancer: Brief Review of Aetiological Studies

As noted above, the aetiology of obesity in the general paediatric population is surprisingly complex and remains incompletely understood despite its apparently simple origin in chronic positive energy balance [17].

One barrier to an improved understanding of the aetiology of obesity in childhood cancer is the need to integrate a diverse array of evidence [17]. The evidence includes physiological studies, which attempt to attribute obesity development to reduced total energy expenditure (energy requirement is determined by total energy expenditure not resting energy expenditure and so it is important to measure the total energy expenditure) and/or increased energy intake [47, 48, 52]; epidemiological studies which attempt to identify behaviours or characteristics of patients or treatments which are associated with or predictive of obesity [17, 37]; mechanistic studies, including studies of genetic predispositions to obesity [53, 54]; intervention studies, which aim to alter a behaviour (or treatment) and examine the impact of the alteration on obesity development.

At present, there appear to be no intervention studies in childhood cancer which have attempted to alter patient behaviour or treatment regimens in order to prevent obesity, though such studies could be very informative in understanding the aetiology of obesity as well as providing valuable practical information which would help prevent and treat obesity. Interventions aimed at reducing sedentary behaviour (table 2) in patients during and after treatment might be the most useful option in preventing many of the harmful sequelae of childhood cancer treatments, including disordered metabolism, impaired bone health, and adverse effects on psychosocial outcomes [46]. Sedentary behaviour is now regarded as a construct which is separate from physical activity, with different determinants and effects [17]. In addition, sedentary behaviour appears to be more modifiable for children and families than physical activity [17]. Intervention studies, preferably multicentre randomised controlled trials focused on modification of sedentary behaviour, should therefore be a priority for future research in obesity associated with childhood cancer, both as a means of understanding the aetiology of obesity [17] and related diseases and as a means of preventing and treating obesity [55].

Energy balance studies have been very helpful in identifying causes of energy imbalance and obesity in ALL. For example, a markedly reduced total energy expenditure, the result of reduced energy expended on physical activity in patients during and after therapy compared to controls, must contribute to excess weight gain and obesity [47, 52]. In one sense, reduced physical activity is therefore a major 'cause' of obesity in ALL, but the underlying cause of reduced physical activity is less clear and might be important to understand when developing interventions aimed at increasing physical activity. Marked reductions in physical activity could occur for a variety of reasons: psychosocial responses to ALL and its treatment might lead to reductions in physical activity and increases in sedentary behaviour; motor impairments, musculoskeletal pathology and/or impairments of exercise capacity might be the underlying 'causes' of reduced levels of physical activity [36, 56, 57], and reduced physical activity might in turn contribute to motor impairment, musculoskeletal pathology, and reduced exercise capacity in a vicious circle.

In summary, energy balance studies have been extremely informative at providing physiological explanations for energy imbalance, particularly if they focus on measurements of total energy expenditure, but such studies cannot provide more fundamental underlying explanations for energy imbalance.

One other limitation to the utility of energy balance studies is when the degree of energy imbalance being experienced by patients is small [17]. Imprecision in the measurement of energy intake is a particular problem when attempting to identify if energy intake makes a contribution to energy imbalance, but even the more accurate and precise measures of energy expenditure may not be adequate if patients are developing obesity gradually, as the result of a small daily energy imbalance of perhaps 50 kcal/day or less [17]. Total energy expenditure studies, and even studies of energy intake, have identified abnormalities in energy balance in ALL successfully because these are so marked, with patients in substantial energy imbalance, at times experiencing abnormally high energy intakes (>250 kcal/day [48]) and/or abnormally low total energy expenditure (reductions of >250 kcal/day relative to controls have been observed in two studies using different methods of measuring total energy expenditure [47, 52]).

Where the rate of energy imbalance is more small and subtle, 'epidemiological' approaches to aetiology may be more informative than energy balance studies [17]. Such studies do not depend on energy balance measures but attempt to identify behaviours, aspects of treatment, or patient characteristics, which are associated with or predictive of obesity [37, 58]. These behaviours or characteristics might be more readily identifiable than the energy imbalances studied by physiological approaches, and should have greater clinical usefulness since they might provide information on features of patients or their treatment which would help either prevent obesity or identify particularly high risk groups within a population of patients. In patients with ALL, though all patients are at high risk of obesity [38], a number of features have been associated consistently with a higher risk of obesity/excess weight gain in 'epidemiological studies', notably early age at diagnosis and gender [37, 58]. Non-modifiable features (age at diagnosis; gender) identified by such studies could be used to identify patients at particularly high risk who might be regarded as priorities for interventions aimed at prevention or treatment of obesity or cardiovascular/metabolic risk factor reduction. In future, genetic studies might also inform such a process by identifying groups with genetic predisposition to obesity and related diseases [53, 54]. Identification of 'risk factors' for obesity development in childhood cancer which were potentially modifiable, such as particular behaviours, would permit targeting of preventive interventions at these factors or behaviours [17, 49].

One important candidate risk factor for obesity in ALL is the rapid growth in adiposity and early 'adiposity rebound' which appears to be a typical consequence of the treatment of childhood obesity [59], and may explain why younger patients with ALL, particularly with onset of the disease during the toddler and preschool years, are at highest risk of obesity. Rapid early growth and adiposity development, such as early adiposity rebound, appears to be a potent risk factor for later obesity more generally [60], though whether the rapid growth is the underlying cause of increased obesity risk or simply a marker of some other cause is unclear [61].

Epidemiological approaches to identifying 'causes' or 'risk factors' for obesity in childhood cancer are likely to continue to be informative, even when retrospective, particularly if sample sizes are large. As noted above, small sample sizes and heterogeneity of patient groups have been typical in the literature and these limitations have hindered our understanding of the aetiology of obesity in childhood cancer [37]. The study (even the retrospective study) of large national or international cohorts would provide a potential solution to this problem, using data from patients treated on similar protocols. Even relatively simple measures of exposures or risk factors (such as patient age) and outcomes (such as BMI SD score) when combined with large sample sizes, have provided very valuable insights into the aetiology of obesity in the past and should continue to do so in the future [17]. If more sophisticated measures of exposures are available such studies would become even more informative. For example, objective and quantitative measurement of physical activity using accelerometry is now practical [17] and has been used to provide novel insights into the causes of impaired bone health in patients treated for ALL [62].

It has been argued that more sophisticated measures of obesity outcome, e.g. more direct measures of body composition such as DEXA, would provide insights not available from the study of simple indices of obesity such as BMI. As noted above, the high diagnostic accuracy of a high BMI for age means that it provides a very good outcome as a simple index of a high fat mass [9, 17]. At lower points in the BMI for age distribution the BMI is less informative of fatness and becomes more limited. Longitudinal study designs which monitor changes in body composition in large cohorts of patients would be helpful in understanding energy balance changes in the 'normal weight' and overweight patient, and a study of this kind in Canadian patients is underway at present [63]. It should be noted however that DEXA alone is not a 'gold standard' in the measurement of paediatric body composition, only multi-component models are gold standards [64, 65], and previous studies with DEXA have found large errors in body composition estimates when compared to multi-component models [66, 67]. However, the high precision of DEXA, particularly suitable for measurement of changes in body composition, its widespread availability, and its added value as a measure of bone health, as noted above, all provide arguments for its cautious use.

The preceding section considered the issue of the size of the average daily energy imbalance being important to determining whether approaches to understanding the aetiology of obesity should be more physiological (energy imbalance research) or more epidemiological (studies of exposures or risk factors). Even in the most-studied of the childhood cancers in terms of obesity research, ALL, the size or rate of energy imbalance being experienced by patients is unclear and has not been estimated or measured. Estimates of the degree of energy imbalance would require measures of changes in body composition over periods of a year or more, with assumptions made in relation to the energetic efficiency of body tissues gained over the year [17]. Such estimates are rare, and have been made for only two cohort studies in the general paediatric population [68, 69], but usefully indicate both how aetiology should be studied and the extent to which lifestyle must change in order to abolish the excessive positive energy balance responsible for obesity [70]. In the USA, such studies suggest that drastic changes in diet and physical activity would be necessary to prevent obesity: with daily energy imbalances typically exceeding 200 kcal/day, prevention of obesity would require substantial changes in both energy intake and total energy expenditure. The generalisability of such findings to populations of children or adolescents being treated for cancer is unclear, but the rate or magnitude of positive energy balance is very marked during and after treatment for ALL and prevention of obesity during the first few years after diagnosis is likely to require drastic changes in lifestyle or treatment.

Preventive interventions in childhood cancer in future should, ideally, be informed by an indication of the magnitude of the energy imbalance which patients are experiencing, and tailor the magnitude of the intervention to the magnitude of the energy imbalance which is likely to be experienced by patients.

Impact of Obesity on Prognosis and Other Outcomes in Childhood Cancer

Table 1 summarises the principal health-related consequences of childhood obesity. These adverse health consequences give particular cause for concern given the high prevalence of obesity in some groups of patients treated for childhood cancer, but an additional concern is that obesity in childhood cancer (and/or the lifestyle and treatment which has caused obesity) might exacerbate other sequelae of childhood cancer such as impairments in bone health, musculoskeletal health, and cardiovascular and metabolic health.

One very recent concern has been the suggestion that obesity might be an adverse prognostic factor in ALL [71]. While this potentially important observation awaits confirmation, there are a number of plausible biological reasons why obesity might compromise the efficacy of treatment [44, 71–73]. In summary, obesity in ALL, and possibly in other malignancies, may become a central issue in prognosis, as well as an important issue in ameliorating 'late effects'.

Potential for Preventive and Treatment Interventions for Obesity during and after Childhood Cancer Treatment

The evidence based on specific interventions for the prevention and treatment of childhood obesity has been repeatedly reviewed systematically and appraised for quality in recent years [2–9] (table 2). While major gaps in the evidence remain, the summarised and appraised evidence to date should provide the starting point in the development of preventive and treatment interventions for obesity in childhood cancer. Good evidence is available on the behaviours which should be targeted in preventive and treatment interventions: sedentary behaviour; physical activity, and diet. There is an increasing and improving evidence base on the issue of *how* to encourage lifestyle change in treatment, as well as a possible role for less traditional obesity therapy such as residential treatments, drug treatments, and bariatric surgery [2–8].

As noted above, interventions aimed at preventing obesity and its sequelae have not been undertaken in childhood cancer, though a few interventions for treatment of hypothalamic obesity have been published [74, 75]. One unresolved issue is the extent to which interventions aimed at preventing or treating obesity in childhood cancer should or could depart from the evidence-based guidance for the general paediatric population. Modifications of prevention and treatment strategies are probably necessary for the specific clinical and family circumstances, but the nature of these modifications remains unclear. Some preventive and treatment interventions, notably promotion of a reduction in sedentary behaviour and increases in physical activity, are likely to have benefits for a wide range of 'late effects' of childhood cancer treatment. Such interventions should be prioritised and their effects on a wide range of outcomes assessed formally, preferably in large, adequately powered and designed, studies, which in practice will probably mean multicentre randomised controlled trials. Given the relatively good understanding of the aetiology and natural history, and the high risk of and from obesity, patients with ALL and possibly tumours in the hypothalamo-pituitary region would appear to be the most pressing priority for intervention studies of this kind. Given the seriousness of the adverse effects of childhood cancer/cancer treatment, the increasing number of childhood cancer survivors, and the range of potential benefits of physical activity which could address many of the adverse effects directly, it is perhaps surprising that no trials based on physical activity promotion (and/or sedentary behaviour reduction) in childhood cancer have yet been published and few if any appear to be underway.

Acknowledgements

The funding for the author's work in ALL was from the UK Leukaemia Research Fund. Other obesity work was funded by grants from the Wellcome Trust, the Scottish Government Health Directorates, Sport Aiding Medical Research for Kids, and the British Heart Foundation.

References

1 Lobstein T, Baur L, Uauy R: Obesity in children and young people: a crisis in public health. Obes Rev 2004;5(suppl 1):4–104.

2 Scottish Intercollegiate Guidelines Network (SIGN) Guideline Number 69: Management of obesity in children and young people: a national clinical guideline. www.sign.ac.uk (accessed Feb 15, 2008).

3 Reilly JJ, Wilson M, Summerbell CD, Wilson DC: Obesity diagnosis, prevention, and treatment: evidence-based answers to common questions. Arch Dis Child 2002;86:392–395.

4 Reilly JJ, Kelnar CJ, Alexander DW, Hacking B, Stewart L, Methven E: Health consequences of obesity. Arch Dis Child 2003;88:748–752.

5 Clinical practice guidelines for the management of overweight and obesity in children and adolescents. www.obesityguidelines.gov.au (accessed Feb 15, 2008).

6 Barlow E, Dietz WH: Obesity evaluation and treatment: Expert Committee recommendations. Pediarics 1998;102:e29–e41.

7 Barlow SE: Expert committee recommendations regarding the prevention, assessment, and treatment of child and adolescent overweight and obesity: summary report. Pediatrics 2007;120: s164–s192.

8 Davis MM, Gance-Cleveland B, Hassink S, Johnson R, Paradis G, Resnicow K: Recommendations for prevention of childhood obesity. Pediatrics 2007;120:s229–s253.

9 Reilly JJ: Diagnostic accuracy of the BMI for age in pediatrics. Int J Obes 2006;30:595–597.

10 Warner JT, Cowan FJ, Dunstan FDJ, Gregory JW: The validity of BMI for the assessment of adiposity in children with disease states. Ann Hum Biol 1997;24:209–215.

11 Cole TJ, Bellizzi MC, Flegal KM, Dietz WH: Establishing a standard definition for child overweight and obesity worldwide: international survey. BMJ 2000;220:1240–1243.

12 Reilly JJ: Assessment of childhood obesity: national reference data or 'international' approach? Obes Res 2002;10:838–840.

13 Yusuf S, Hawken S, Ounpuu S, Bautista L, Fransozi MG, Commerford P, Lang CC, Ruboldt Z, Onen CL, Lisheig L, Tanomsup S, Wangai P, Razak F, Sharma AM, Annand SS, INTERHEART Study Investigators: Obesity and the risk of myocardial infarction in 27,000 participants from 52 countries: a case-control study. Lancet 2005; 366: 1640–1649.

14 Freedman DS, Kahn HS, Mei Z, Grummer-Strawn LM, Dietz WH, Srinivasan SR, Berenson GS: Relation of BMI and waist-to height ratio to cardiovascular disease risk factors in children and adolescents: the Bogalusa Heart Study. Am J Clin Nutr 2007;86:33–40.

15 Ng VW, Kong APS, Chow Choi K, Ozaki R, Wong GWK, So WY, Tong PCY, Sung RYT, Yu Y, Chan MHM, Ho CS, Lam CWK, Chan JCN: BMI and waist circumference in predicting cardiovascular risk factor clustering in Chinese adolescents. Obesity 2007;15:494–503.

16 Garnett SP, Baur LA, Srinivasan S, Lee JW, Cowell CT: BMI and waist circumference in mid-childhood and adverse cardiovascular risk clustering in adolescence. Am J Clin Nutr 2007;86:549–555.

17 Reilly JJ, Ness AR, Sherriff A: Epidemiologic and physiologic approaches to understanding the etiology of pediatric obesity: finding the needle in the haystack. Pediatr Res 2007;61:646–652.

18 Whitaker RC: Preventing pediatric obesity: four behaviors to target. Arch Pediatr Adolesc Med 2003;157:725–727.

19 Schwimmer JB, Deutsch R, Kahen T, Lavine JE, Stanley C, Behling C: Prevalence of fatty liver in children and adolescents. Pediatrics 2006;118: 1388–1393.

20 Schwimmer JB, Burwinkle TM, Varni JW: Health-related quality of life of severely obese children and adolescents. JAMA 2003;289:1813–1819.

21 Hughes AR, Farewell K, Harris D, Reilly JJ: Quality of life in a clinical sample of obese children. Int J Obes 2007;31:39–44.

22 Lawlor DA, Martin RM, Gunnell D, Galobardes B, Ebrahim S, Sandhu J, Ben-Shlomo Y, McCarron P, Davey-Smith G: Associations of BMI measured in childhood, adolescence, and young adulthood with risk of ischemic heart disease and stroke: findings from 3 historical cohort studies. Am J Clin Nutr 2006;63:767–773.
23 Baker JL, Olsen LW, Sorensen TI: Childhood BMI and the risk of coronary heart disease in adulthood. N Engl J Med 2007;357:2329–2337.
24 Viner RM, Cole TJ: Adult socio-economic, educational, social, and psychological outcomes of childhood obesity: national birth cohort study. BMJ 2005;330:1354–1358.
25 Freedman DS, Khan LK, Serdula MK, Dietz WH, Srinivasan SR, Berenson GS: Racial differences in the tracking of childhood BMI to adulthood. Obes Res 2005;13:928–935.
26 Freedman DS, Khan LK, Serdula MK, Dietz WH, Srinivasan SR, Berenson GS: The relation of childhood BMI to adult adiposity: Bogalusa Heart Study. Pediatrics 2005;115:22–27.
27 Summerbell CD, Ashton V, Campbell KJ, Edmunds L, Kelly S, Waters E: Interventions for treating obesity in children. Cochrane Database Syst Rev 2005;3:CD001872.
28 Summerbelll CD, Waters E, Edmunds LD, Kelly S, Brown T, Campbell KJ: Interventions for preventing obesity in children. Cochrane Database Syst. Rev 2005;3:CD001871.
29 Hughes AR, Stewart L, Chapple J, McColl JH, Donaldson M, Kelnar CJ, Zabihollah M, Ahmed F, Reilly JJ: Randomized, controlled trial of a best-practice individualized behavioral program for treatment of childhood overweight: Scottish Childhood Overweight Treatment Trial (SCOTT). Pediatrics 2008;121:e539–e46.
30 Edwards C, Nicholls D, Croker H, Van Zyl S, Viner R, Wardle J: Family-based behavioural treatment of obesity: acceptability and effectiveness in the UK. Eur J Clin Nutr 2006;60:587–592.
31 Reilly JJ: Tackling the obesity epidemic: new approaches. Arch Dis Child 2006;91:721–726.
32 Savoye M, Shaw M, Dziura J, Tamborlane WV, Rose P Guandalini C, Goldberg R, Burgert TS, Cali AM, Weiss R, Caprio S: Effects of a weight management program on body composition and metabolic parameters in overweight children: a randomized controlled trial. JAMA 2007;297:-2697–2704.
33 Reinehr T, Andler W: Changes in the atherogenic risk factor profile according to degree of weight loss. Arch Dis Child 2004;89:419–422.
34 Stewart L, Hughes AR, Chapple J, Poustie V, Reilly JJ: The patient journey in childhood obesity treatment: a qualitative study. Arch Dis Child 2008;93:35–39.
35 Murtagh J, Dixey R, Rudolf M: A qualitative investigation into the levers and barriers to weight loss in children: opinions of obese children. Arch Dis Child 2006;9:920–923.
36 Warner JT: Body composition, exercise and energy expenditure in survivors of acute lymphoblastic leukemia. Pediatr Blood Cancer 2008;50: 456–461.
37 Brouwer CAJ, Gietema JA, Kamps WA, de Vries EGE, Postma A: Changes in body composition after childhood cancer treatment: impact on future health status – a review. Crit Rev Oncol Hematol 2007;63:32–46.
38 Gregory JW, Reilly JJ: Body composition and obesity; in Wallace H, Green D (eds): Late Effects of Childhood Cancer. London, Arnold, 2004, pp 147–161.
39 Oeffinger KC, Mertens AC, Sklar CA, Yasui Y, Fears T, Stovall M, Vik TA, Inskip PD, Robinson LL: Obesity in adult survivors of childhood ALL. J Clin Oncol 2003;21:1350–1365.
40 Dickerman JD: The late effects of childhood cancer therapy. Pediatrics 2007;119:554–568.
41 Reilly JJ: Descriptive epidemiology and health consequences of childhood obesity. Best Prac Res Clin Endocrinol Metab 2005;19:327–341.
42 Levine RS, Feltblower RG, Connor AM, Robinson M, Rudolf MC: Monitoring trends in childhood obesity: a simple school-based model. Public Health 2008;122:255–260.
43 Reilly JJ, Weir J, McColl JH, Gibson BES: Prevalence of protein-energy malnutrition at diagnosis in children treated for acute lymphoblastic leukemia. J Pediatr Gastroenterol Nutr 1999;29:194–197.
44 Rogers PC, Meacham LR, Oeffinger KC: Obesity in pediatric oncology. Pediatr Blood Cancer 2005;45:881–891.
45 Wells JCK, Fewtrell MS: Is body composition important for paediatricians? Arch Dis Child 2008;93:168–172.
46 Janiszewski PM, Oeffinger KM, Church TS, Dunn AL, Eshelman DA, Victor RG, Brooks S, Turoff AJ, Sinclair E, Murray JC, Bashare L, Ross R: Abdominal obesity, liver fat, and muscle composition in survivors of childhood acute lymphoblastic leukemia. J Clin Endocrinol Metab 2007;92:3816–3821.

47 Reilly JJ, Ventham JC, Ralston JM, Donaldson M, Gibson BES: Reduced energy expenditure in pre-obese children treated for acute lymphoblastic leukemia. Pediatr Res 1998;44:557–562.

48 Reilly JJ, Brougham M, Montgomery C, Gibson BES: Effect of glucocorticoid therapy on energy intake in children treated for acute lymphoblastic leukemia. J Clin Endocrinol Metab 2001;86:3742–3745.

49 Reilly JJ, Armstrong J, Dorosty AR, Emmett PM, Rogers IS, Steer C, Ness AR, Sherriff A: Early life risk factors for childhood obesity: cohort study. BMJ 2005;330:1357–1361.

50 Hoffman HJ, De Silva M, Humphreys RP: Aggressive surgical management of craniopharyngiomas in children. J Neurosurg 1992;76:47–52.

51 De Vile CJ, Grant DB, Hayward RD: Obesity in childhood craniopharyngioma: relation to post-operative hypothalamic damage shown by magnetic resonance imaging. J Clin Endocrinol Metab 1996;81:2734–2737.

52 Warner JT, Bell W, Webb DKH, Gregory JW: Daily energy expenditure and physical activity in survivors of childhood malignancy Pediatr Res 1998;43:607–613.

53 Ross JA, Oeffinger KC, Davies SM, Mertens AC, Larger EK, Kiffmeyer WR, Sklar CA, Stovall M, Yasui Y, Robison LL: Genetic variation in the leptin receptor gene and obesity in survivors of childhood acute lymphoblastic leukemia. J Clin Oncol 2004;22:3558–3562.

54 Frayling TM, Timpson NJ, Weedon MN, Hattersley AT, McCarthy MI: A common variant in the FTO gene is associated with BMI and predisposes to childhood and adult obesity. Science 2007;373: 47–51.

55 White J, Flohr JA, Winter SS, Vener J, Feinaver LR, Ransdell LB: Potential benefits of physical activity for children with acute lymphoblastic leukemia. Pediatr Rehab 2005;8:53–58.

56 Oeffinger KC: Are survivors of ALL at increased risk of cardiovascular disease? Pediatr Blood Cancer 2008;50:462–467.

57 Ness KK, Baker JS, Dengel DR, Youngren N, Sibley S, Mertens AC, Gurney JG: Body composition, muscle strength deficits, and mobility limitations in adult survivors of childhood ALL. Pediatr Blood Cancer 2007;49:975–981.

58 Reilly JJ: Energy balance and its measurement in childhood disease. Pediatr Blood Cancer 2008;50: 452–455.

59 Reilly JJ, Kelly A, Ness P, Dorosty AR, Wallace WHB, Gibson BES, Emmett PM: Premature adiposity rebound in children treated for acute lymphoblastic leukaemia. J Clin Endocrinol Metab 2001;86:2775–2778.

60 Baird J, Fisher D, Lucas P, Kleijnen J, Roberts H, Law C. Being big or growing fast: systematic review of size and growth in infancy and later obesity. BMJ 2005;331:929–932.

61 Cole TJ: Children grow and horses race: is the adiposity rebound a critical period for later obesity? BMC Pediatr 2004;12:4–6.

62 Tillmann V, Darlington AS, Eiser C, Bishop NJ, Davies HA: Male sex and low physical activity are associated with reduced spine bone mineral obesity in survivors of childhood ALL. J Bone Mineral Res 2002;17:1033–1080.

63 Rogers PC, Melnick SJ, Ladas EJ, Halton JH, Baillargeon J, Sucks N: Children's Oncology Group (COG) Nutrition Committee. Pediatr Blood Cancer 2008;50(suppl):447–451.

64 Wells JC, Fewtrell MF: Measuring body composition. Arch Dis Child 2006;91:612–617.

65 Reilly JJ: Assessment of body composition in infants and children. Nutrition 1998;14:821–825.

66 Williams JE, Wells JC, Wilson CM, Haroun D, Lucas A, Fewtrell MS: Evaluation of Lunar Prodigy dual-energy X-ray absorptiometry for assessing body composition in healthy persons and patients by comparison with the criterion 4-compartment model. Am J Clin Nutr 2006;83:1047–1054.

67 Shypaillo RJ, Butte NF, Ellis KJ: DEXA: can it be used as a criterion reference for body fat measurements in children ? Obesity 2008;16:457–462.

68 Butte NF, Ellis KT: Comment on 'Obesity and the environment: where do we go from here?' Science 2003;301:598.

69 Wang YC, Gortmaker SC, Sobol AM, Kantz KM: Estimating the energy gap amongst US children. Pediatrics 2006;118:e1721–e1833.

70 Butte NF, Christiensen E, Sorensen TI: Energy imbalance underlying the development of childhood obesity. Obesity 2007;15:3056–3066.

71 Butturini AM, Dorey FJ, Large BJ, Henry DW, Gaynon PS, FU C, Franklin J, Siegel SE, Seibel NL, Rogers PC, Sather H, Trigg M, Bleger WA, Carroll WL: Obesity and outcome in pediatric ALL. J Clin Oncol 2007;25:2063–2069.

72 JJ Reilly, Workman P: Normalisation of anti-cancer drug dosage using body weight and surface area. Cancer Chemother Pharmacol 1993;32:411–418.

73 JJ Reilly, Workman P: Is body composition an important variable in the pharmacokinetics of anti-cancer drugs? Cancer Chemother Pharmacol 1994;34:3–13.
74 Danielsson P, Janson A, Norgren S, Marcus C: Impact sibutramine therapy in children with hypothalamic obesity or obesity with aggravating syndromes. J Clin Endocrinol Metab 2007;92: 4101–4106.
75 Lustig RH, Hinds PS, Ringwald-Smith K, Christensen RK, Kaste SC, Schreiber RE, Rai SN, Lensing SY, Wa S, Xiong X: Ocreotide therapy for pediatric hypothalamic obesity. J Clin Endocrinol Metab 2003;88:2586–1592.

John J. Reilly
Professor of Paediatric Energy Metabolism
Division of Developmental Medicine, Yorkhill Hospitals, University of Glasgow
1st Floor Tower QMH
Glasgow G3 8SJ (UK)
Tel. +44 141 201 0710, Fax +44 141 201 0674, E-Mail jjr2y@clinmed.gla.ac.uk

Wallace WHB, Kelnar CJH (eds): Endocrinopathy after Childhood Cancer Treatment.
Endocr Dev. Basel, Karger, 2009, vol 15, pp 59–76

Metabolic Disorders

John W. Gregory

Department of Child Health, Wales School of Medicine, Cardiff University, Cardiff, UK

Abstract

Adult survivors of childhood cancer, particularly brain tumours and acute lymphoblastic leukaemia demonstrate evidence of increased rates of metabolic complications and cardiovascular disease in later life. Evidence is accumulating that risk factors for these complications include obesity, physical inactivity, lipid abnormalities, insulin resistance and development of the metabolic syndrome. Cranial radiotherapy-induced growth hormone deficiency, other direct adverse effects of radiotherapy and anthracycline-induced left ventricular dysfunction are clearly identified risk factors for developing these complications. Growth hormone replacement, where appropriate, has been of some benefit in reducing the prevalence of metabolic complications in some long-term survivors. In others, it is clear that multidisciplinary interventions will need to be developed which focus on modifying aspects of lifestyle including increasing levels of habitual physical activity, improving diet and prevention of smoking along with the use of lipid-lowering medication.

The Metabolic Syndrome

The term 'metabolic syndrome' or 'syndrome X' has been applied to a clustering of abnormalities which predispose to the risk in later life of cardiovascular disease [1, 2] and represents one of the major worldwide challenges to public health. The association of hypertension, insulin resistance, hyperglycaemia, increased serum triglyceride and low high-density lipoprotein (HDL) cholesterol concentrations was highlighted by Reaven [3] in 1988. Subsequently, other associations have been reported including obesity [4], microalbuminuria [5], abnormalities in fibrinolysis and coagulation [6] and polycystic ovarian disease [7].

Aetiology

The aetiology of the metabolic syndrome remains unclear though insulin resistance was initially proposed to play a key role [3]. Others have suggested that visceral obesity and the association of an increased waist circumference with elevated plasma triglyceride concentrations are important risk factors for the syndrome [8]. Probably, several factors are involved including those related to changes in lifestyle [9].

Definitions

Regardless of the aetiology, defining the metabolic syndrome has been controversial leading to difficulties interpreting the implications of published data [10]. The situation is also complicated by ethnic differences that mean for example that people of Asian origin are at risk of type 2 diabetes at lower levels of adiposity than are those of European origins [11]. Furthermore, in childhood, there are no agreed definitions as to what constitutes the metabolic syndrome, though obesity in childhood is known to increase the risk of cardiovascular disease through adolescence into young adulthood [12, 13]. The International Diabetes Federation has now published suggested definitions for the metabolic syndrome [10, 14] which are summarised in table 1.

Whilst there has been considerable debate about the precise definition such that prevalence and predictive values vary widely depending on the definition used [15], there is little argument that the components represent a maladjustment of human physiology to a changing nutritional environment and pattern of energy expenditure [16], usually a combination of excess energy intake for the reducing levels of physical activity.

Implications

Although the prognosis for individuals with the metabolic syndrome will vary depending on the definition used, in adult life, there are clearly significant adverse implications for longevity. For example, using the World Health Organisation definition [17], a Scandinavian study has shown in 35- to 70-year-olds a threefold increased risk of coronary heart disease or stroke and a sixfold increase in cardiovascular mortality during a near 7-year follow-up period [1]. Others have shown similar increases in both cardiovascular disease and all-cause mortality in men with the metabolic syndrome even in the absence of baseline cardiovascular disease and diabetes which affects so many of these individuals when diagnosed [2].

Prevention

There is increasing evidence that lifestyle advice promoting increasing levels of physical activity and weight loss may be beneficial in preventing the metabolic syndrome [18]. Physical activity, weight loss and diet have been shown to have short-term benefits on some of the individual components of the metabolic syndrome [2]. Recent randomised controlled trials in the general population are

Table 1. International Diabetes Federation definition of at-risk groups and of metabolic syndrome

Age 6–10 years • Obesity ≥90th percentile as assessed by waist circumference • Metabolic syndrome cannot be diagnosed, but further measurements should be made if family history of metabolic syndrome, type 2 diabetes mellitus, dyslipidaemia, cardiovascular disease, hypertension or obesity
Age 10–16 years • Obesity ≥90th percentile (or adult cut-off if lower) as assessed by waist circumference • Triglycerides ≥1.7 mmol/l • HDL-cholesterol <1.03 mmol/l • Blood pressure ≥130 mm Hg systolic or ≥85 mm Hg diastolic • Glucose ≥5.6 mmol/l (oral glucose tolerance test recommended) or known type 2 diabetes mellitus
Age >16 years • Increased waist circumference (see ethnic-specific table [10]) Plus any two: • Triglycerides ≥1.7 mmol/l • HDL-cholesterol <1.03 mmol/l in men, <1.29 mmol/l in women • Blood pressure ≥130 mm Hg systolic or ≥85 mm Hg diastolic • Glucose ≥5.6 mmol/l (oral glucose tolerance test strongly recommended but not necessary to define the presence of the syndrome) • Previously diagnosed type 2 diabetes

showing that lifestyle interventions can have encouraging results. For example, by comparison with unstructured advice given by family physicians, a general recommendation-based programme of lifestyle intervention carried out by trained professionals has been shown to be effective in reducing multiple metabolic and associated inflammatory abnormalities in middle-aged adults [19].

Risk Factors for Metabolic Disorders in Survivors of Childhood Malignancy

Whereas in the general population, the metabolic syndrome may represent a maladaptive response to energy surplus caused by either genetic influences or effects of the in utero environment [16], in survivors of childhood cancer it is more likely that direct tumour effects or consequences of the curative therapy have led to the increased risk that these individuals experience. Potential mechanisms (fig. 1) which may predispose to overweight and metabolic complications have been identified mostly in those who have undergone therapy for intracranial tumours [20, 21] or cranial radiotherapy for acute lymphoblastic leukaemia (ALL) [22–25].

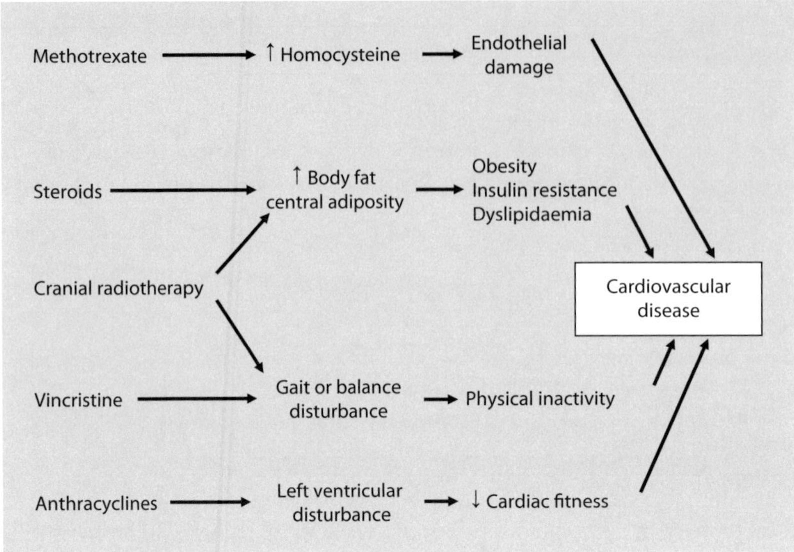

Fig. 1. Risk factors for the development of cardiovascular disease. Adapted from Oeffinger [84].

These include steroid treatment during acute treatment, tumour-, surgery- or radiotherapy-induced hypothalamo-pituitary axis damage, direct damage to the satiety centre in the ventromedial hypothalamus [21], leptin insensitivity [26, 27], growth hormone deficiency [25], cardiorespiratory complications [28–30] and impaired physical activity [31].

Obesity

Obesity is a well-recognised complication of the treatment of certain childhood malignancies, particularly ALL [24, 32–36]. A Canadian study [35] which evaluated the body mass indices of 441 childhood and teenage cancer survivors at a median age of 14.7 years showed that 20.9% were overweight and 10.9% obese. Whilst it was concluded that the prevalence of overweight for the group as a whole was no greater than that for the general population, male survivors of ALL had an increased risk (odds ratio (OR) 1.55; 95% confidence interval (CI) 1.03–2.52; p = 0.04). A similar but much larger study has also been undertaken in the USA, evaluating the body mass indices this time of 7,195 adults who had survived at least 5 years from the treatment of cancer in childhood. Again, this demonstrated that survivors of ALL had demonstrated an increased risk of obesity (OR 1.5, 95% CI 1.2–1.8 and OR 1.2, 95% CI 1.0–1.5 for males and females, respectively) [34]. The use of body mass indices to identify obesity in survivors of childhood ALL may be of limited value due to the many influences that may affect the relationship between height, weight and body composition [37]. More objective measures of body composition including measurement of skin-fold thicknesses and dual energy X-ray absorptiometry have confirmed evidence of increased adiposity in this group [22] compared with reference populations even when body mass indices are not increased [38].

Children with brain tumours, especially surgically operated craniopharyngioma are at a high risk of 'hypothalamic' obesity [39, 40], a severe form of obesity which seems poorly responsive to most therapies and a consequence of damage to the hypothalamus [41]. A large cohort (156 children with primary brain tumours) at one centre in the USA have been studied retrospectively to identify risk factors for the development of obesity [21]. Over an approximate 11-year period of follow-up from diagnosis, these included younger age at diagnosis, a radiation dose range of 51–72 Gy to the hypothalamus even after exclusion of hypothalamic and thalamic tumours, the presence of any endocrinopathy, location of the tumour at the hypothalamus, extent of surgery and the presence of specific tumours (craniopharyngioma, pilocytic astrocytoma and medulloblastoma). These findings largely suggest that hypothalamic damage, whether caused by the tumour, radiotherapy or surgery, is the main cause of obesity in children with brain tumours. By contrast, however, an even larger North American multicentre study of 921 adults aged 20–45 years did not demonstrate a body mass index distribution that differed from the population norms, though in females, a younger age at diagnosis and radiation to the hypothalamo-pituitary axis were associated with an increased risk of obesity [42].

Physical Inactivity

Regardless of the cause, relative physical inactivity may predispose to increased body weight and metabolic disturbance. Self-report questionnaires show that adult survivors of childhood ALL are more likely to be inactive (OR 1.74, 95% CI 1.56–1.94) compared with the general population and that those who received cranial irradiation >20 Gy were at particular risk [43]. A large-scale questionnaire study of long-term survivors of childhood cancer shows that compared with siblings, survivors particularly of brain (26.6%) and bone cancer (36.9%) were more likely to report limitations in physical performances (OR 1.8, 95% CI 1.7–2.0) including those linked to vigorous and moderate activities [44]. Objective measurements in survivors of childhood leukaemia have confirmed reduced levels of physical activity [31] and decreased energy expended on habitual physical activity [45]. For example, in a study of 34 such patients, mean total daily energy expenditure and levels of physical activity measured by continuous heart rate recording were both reduced by approximately 29% compared with control subjects. Children surviving other childhood malignancies had values similar to controls [31]. Further studies in this group have demonstrated that peak oxygen consumption in response to maximal levels of exercise, which is a measure of aerobic physical fitness, is reduced and correlated with measures of physical activity [46]. Others have confirmed in a meta-analysis of several studies that physical fitness is decreased in the longer term in older survivors [47].

Reduced muscle mass, metabolic function and strength may impair the capacity to undertake physical activity. Leg weakness has been demonstrated in a small group of children during treatment for ALL [48] and also in a larger group of adolescent and young adult survivors [49]. Adult survivors of childhood ALL have been shown to have reduced lean body mass, quadriceps strength and mobility as measured by the time taken to stand up and walk a few steps from an armchair before returning to sit down and the distance they could walk in 2 min [50]. In the female study subjects, both cranial irradiation and growth hormone deficiency were associated with strength deficits suggesting a possible causal relationship [49, 50]. However, others have shown decreased trunk muscle strength and performance in a varied group of survivors of childhood cancer but have failed to show any relationship between these outcomes and previous cranial irradiation or the presence of growth hormone deficiency [51] though this may partly reflect the heterogenous nature of the patient group. Nevertheless, young age at diagnosis and serum testosterone concentrations in male survivors were shown to be associated with measures of muscle strength and performance. Testosterone is known to have a powerful anabolic action stimulating muscle protein synthesis and muscle mass in adults [52].

Adverse effects on cardiac function from chemotherapy may impair an individual's capacity to undertake physical exercise. Patients treated for childhood ALL have been demonstrated to have higher heart rate levels at rest and at low levels of exercise suggesting the possibility that chemotherapy-induced toxicity was affecting augmentation of stroke volume [31]. Anthracyclines have long been known to have adverse effects on cardiac function particularly left ventricular structure and function [28, 53]. Recent long-term studies have shown that chronic progressive cardiac dysfunction persists for many years after treatment leading to an inadequate ventricular mass with a chronic after-load excess associated with a progressive contractile deficit and possibly reduced cardiac output with a restrictive cardiomyopathy [54].

In addition to the late effects of anthracyclines on cardiac function, radiation of the mediastinum has also been reported to have a range of adverse effects on cardiovascular function including coronary artery disease, pericarditis, cardiomyopathy and valvular disease [29]. These complications may all give rise to fatigue, dyspnoea on exertion, limited exercise capacity and levels of physical activity. The greatest risk of developing these adverse effects is seen in those receiving higher total doses of radiation (>35–40 Gy/day), higher fractionated doses (>2.0 Gy/day), having greater volumes of heart exposed, at a younger age of exposure and following longer periods of follow-up after irradiation.

The lung is one of the most radiation-sensitive organs in the body influenced by the volume of tissue irradiated, the total dose received and fractionation scheduling. Radiation in childhood has been shown to reduce lung function and dynamic lung compliance, possibly due to failure of alveolar development, resulting from impaired cell proliferation. Furthermore, several chemotherapeutic agents are known to produce pulmonary toxicity. By comparison with siblings, survivors report increased rates over more than 5 years from treatment of childhood cancer of lung fibrosis, recurrent pneumonia, chronic cough, pleurisy, use of supplemental oxygen, abnormalities of the chest wall, exercise-induced shortness of breath and bronchitis [30]. Risk factors for such complications include chest irradiation and exposure to bleomycin, cyclophosphamide, busulphan, lomustine or carmustine. Pulmonary complications such as these are also likely to impair exercise capacity and levels of physical activity.

Radiotherapy and Endocrine Dysfunction
It seems likely that of those individuals previously treated for ALL, it is those who have previously been treated with cranial radiotherapy who are most likely to become overweight with those receiving larger doses being at greatest risk. This increase in body mass indices largely occurs whilst undergoing active treatment for the leukaemia with little further increase thereafter [24]. A similar study of the body mass indices of 1,765 adult survivors of childhood ALL has shown that those who received cranial radiation doses of <20 Gy have an increased risk of obesity (OR 2.59, 95% CI 1.88–3.55, and OR 1.86, 95% CI 1.33–2.57, for females and males, respectively) and that this risk was greatest for girls treated under the age of 4 years [25]. Why the latter group should be at greater risk is unclear but may partly relate to the effects of cranial radiotherapy producing earlier onset of puberty [55, 56] and reduced final height [57].

It has been proposed that the greater sensitivity of the younger brain to adverse effects of cranial radiotherapy are likely to be secondary to disturbances of the hypothalamo-pituitary axis leading to growth hormone deficiency or leptin resistance. Cranial radiotherapy has long been known to cause growth hormone deficiency. Studies of spontaneous 24-hour growth hormone profiles in adult survivors of cranial irradiation for non-pituitary tumours in childhood show a reduction in all amplitude-related measurements, increased secretory disorderliness but preserved pulsatility and diurnal variation [58]. In adults, growth hormone deficiency has been shown to be associated with obesity [59, 60] and adult survivors of childhood ALL are known to be at an increased risk of growth hormone deficiency [61]. However, data relating evidence of growth hormone deficiency to obesity in adult survivors of childhood cancer are contradictory with some studies showing an association (50 survivors including 28 with ALL) [62] and others not (90 survivors including 28 with ALL) [63]. Furthermore, the fact that some studies have shown that body mass indices largely increase only during active treatment when most individuals are able to produce normal amounts of growth hormone [64] suggests that these early changes in body composition are unlikely to be mediated by growth hormone deficiency. Nevertheless, ongoing growth hormone deficiency may play a role in the maintenance of increased adiposity once established [24].

Not only is growth hormone deficiency known to be associated with abnormalities in body composition but there is good evidence that adults with growth hormone deficiency are at markedly increased risk of cardiovascular disease. A retrospective study of individuals with hypopituitarism has shown a risk of cardiovascular mortality that was twice that of age- and gender-matched controls despite appropriate replacement of other hormone deficiencies [65]. Cerebrovascular mortality is also increased and presents at a younger age [66]. Growth hormone deficiency is also associated with a range of metabolic abnormalities including increased total cholesterol, low-density lipoprotein (LDL) cholesterol, apolipoprotein B, lipoprotein [a] and triglyceride levels, reduced HDL cholesterol, impaired glucose tolerance and insulin resistance [60]. Whether long-term replacement of growth hormone in these patients prevents premature atherosclerosis leading to a reduction in cardiovascular morbidity and mortality remains to be shown.

Insulin resistance following bone marrow transplantation is also common and in a cohort of young adult survivors, hypogonadism is associated with hyperinsulinaemia [67]. It has been speculated by these authors that a combination of growth hormone deficiency and hypogonadism leads to cellular atrophy in the target organ, predisposing to the development of metabolic risk factors. More recently, others have confirmed evidence that total body irradiation-conditioning for bone marrow transplant, abdominal obesity and untreated hypogonadism are major independent risk factors for developing metabolic complications in survivors of childhood cancer [68]. Steroid treatment has also been suggested as a risk factor through its effects on body composition [69]. However, a much larger study of ALL subjects who had reached final height suggests that cranial radiotherapy rather than steroid treatment during childhood ALL is principally related to longer term risks of obesity [24].

An alternative explanation for radiation-induced obesity may be an injurious effect on centres within the brain that regulate eating and body composition through the development of so-called ‘leptin resistance’ [70, 71]. Leptin is a peptide secreted by adipocytes which stimulates leptin receptors in the ventromedial hypothalamus leading to decreased food intake and increased energy expenditure [72, 73]. Leptin concentrations increase in proportion to increasing body fat stores and are thought to be one of several signals involved in regulating energy balance with body energy stores through largely central mechanisms. Studies have evaluated the possible role of resistance to leptin being responsible for obesity in survivors of childhood leukaemia. In a cohort of 32 adult survivors who received cranial irradiation, increased leptin levels, by comparison with age- and body mass index-adjusted controls in those with abnormalities of growth hormone secretion [70] suggest that hyperleptinaemia might be a consequence of radiation-induced hypothalamic damage or growth hormone deficiency. Subsequently, polymorphisms in the leptin receptor gene have been shown to be associated with obesity in females treated with >20 Gy cranial radiotherapy but not male survivors of leukaemia [26]. However, a later study in a cohort of subjects undergoing chemotherapy for 2 years following diagnosis also showed increasing serum leptin concentrations even after adjustment for their excess adiposity. As this cohort did not receive radiotherapy and demonstrated growth patterns unlikely to suggest evolving growth hormone deficiency, the findings suggest that other mechanisms including a consequence of glucocorticoid treatment may be involved [27].

Metabolic Disorders following Treatment of Childhood Cancer

Long-term survivors of childhood malignancy have long been known to be at increased risk of cardiovascular disease. A UK analysis of 738 deaths in a cohort of 4,082 survivors (at least 5 years out) of childhood cancer showed a fivefold excess of deaths from cardiovascular causes, with those from myocardial infarction and cerebrovascular accidents being the most frequent [74]. A similar increase in mortality and ischaemic heart disease has been reported from a North American study [75]. Whilst direct adverse effects of thoracic radiotherapy and chemotherapy on the heart may account for some of the findings, a study in 1996 of a relatively small heterogenous group of survivors of childhood cancer showed they had increased weight, fat mass, fasting plasma glucose and insulin concentrations with decreased serum HDL cholesterol and a reduced HDL to total cholesterol ratio by comparison with age-matched controls, findings which were thought to be characteristic of the 'metabolic syndrome' [62]. Even after adjustment for their increased relative weight, survivors had evidence of an increased risk of metabolic abnormalities suggesting that increased relative weight is not the only contributor to these findings. The authors postulated that growth hormone deficiency may play a partial role in the evolution of these biochemical abnormalities [76] and that given the central role of the liver in carbohydrate, lipid and insulin metabolism, the hepatotoxic effects of chemotherapy may play an additional role.

Survivors of Brain Tumours

Subsequent studies have confirmed an increased risk of developing markers of the metabolic syndrome in survivors of specific groups of childhood cancer. A controlled study in survivors from childhood brain cancer has shown that in their mid 20s, they have an increased blood pressure, waist-hip ratio, cholesterol/HDL ratio, LDL cholesterol and apolipoprotein B levels and lower HDL cholesterol and that some of these metabolic markers were most abnormal in those who experienced absolute growth hormone deficiency [77]. The relationship between these risk factors for cardiovascular disease and premature atherosclerosis was studied by measurement of the walls of large peripheral arteries using high resolution ultrasound. This showed that the carotid bulb intima media thickness was increased in survivors though other segments of the carotid artery were similar in thickness to controls perhaps reflecting the small sample size of this study. Nevertheless, the authors concluded that these findings may predate the development of symptomatic atherosclerosis.

Survivors of Acute Lymphoblastic Leukaemia

Similar findings have been shown in cohorts of young adult survivors of childhood ALL. A small study of 26 subjects showed that 62% had at least one cardiovascular risk factor (obesity, dyslipidaemia, increased blood pressure or insulin resistance) related to their cancer treatment with 30% having more than two [78]. Thirty-eight percent of the cohort had received cranial irradiation and serum insulin-like growth factor-1 (IGF-1) concentrations were inversely correlated with common carotid artery wall intima media thickness which is thought to be an intermediate marker of cardiovascular disease. Others have shown similar associations between surviving ALL with cranial radiotherapy and increased abdominal and liver fat, insulin resistance and dyslipidaemia with IGF-1 levels being inversely related to the amounts of fat [79]. Although the value of serum IGF-1 as a marker of growth hormone deficiency has been questioned, this finding lends support to the possible role that growth hormone deficiency may play in the frequency of metabolic abnormalities seen in survivors of childhood malignancy. A larger study of 44 adult survivors of childhood ALL of whom 91% were growth hormone deficient confirmed a high incidence of abnormal body composition and dyslipidaemia [80]. The strong correlations between the stimulated peak growth hormone concentration and several cardiovascular risk factors lends weight to the importance of growth hormone deficiency in predisposing to these metabolic abnormalities, a finding supported by others [81] with evidence that women in particular are at greatest risk [20]. A study by Link et al. [80] has also shown raised fibrinogen levels in survivors, a finding also associated with growth hormone deficiency. Raised fibrinogen together with an increased waist-hip ratio and lipid abnormalities links thrombogenesis and atherogenesis and is an independent risk factor for cardiovascular disease at least as important as blood pressure and lipid levels.

Although the above studies largely suggest that cranial irradiation and growth hormone deficiency are key steps in the increased risk of developing complications following treatment of childhood ALL, recent studies have also shown that individuals treated for ALL with chemotherapy alone also demonstrate an increased risk of the metabolic syndrome. A Greek study showed that compared with national prevalence values for the metabolic syndrome in young adults, a twofold increased risk occurred in those who received chemotherapy alone compared with a fivefold increase in those who also received cranial irradiation [82]. It is thought that dysfunction of the vascular epithelium is an early step in the development of cardiovascular disease. Adult survivors of ALL have also been shown to have reduced endothelial-dependent flow-mediated dilatation whether they received chemotherapy alone or chemotherapy with cranial irradiation [83]. The findings of the study suggest that this was due solely to chemotherapy-induced endothelial dysfunction rather than a decline in arterial smooth muscle function. Whether this finding was due to chemotherapy-induced apoptosis of vascular endothelial cells or a consequence of elevate plasma triglyceride concentrations is unknown. Another growth hormone-independent mechanism which has recently been postulated to increase the risk of cardiovascular disease in survivors of ALL therapy is the evidence that methotrexate induces elevations in plasma homocysteine. Homocysteine is known to directly impair endothelial function and promote atherogenesis by facilitating oxidative injury on the vascular endothelium leading to an inflammatory response [84].

Survivors of Bone Marrow Transplantation

Young adult survivors of childhood malignancy who have undergone bone marrow transplantation are at a particularly high risk of metabolic abnormalities. A large self-report survey [85] of 1,089 survivors of haematopoietic cell transplantation who had survived at least 2 years demonstrates, by comparison with siblings, a 3.65 times (95% CI 1.82–7.32) greater prevalence of diabetes and a 2.06 times (95% CI 1.39–3.04) increased risk of hypertension. There was a higher risk of diabetes in those who had undergone allogenic transplantation compared with autologous recipients and in those who had undergone total body irradiation in their conditioning regimens raising the possible role of inflammatory- and cytokine-mediated mechanisms contributing to the development of insulin resistance. This group reported a low prevalence of adverse cardiovascular outcomes perhaps reflecting their relatively young age. More objective studies in a cohort of 23 such survivors, mostly given bone marrow transplantation following treatment of previous childhood ALL, show that 52% had insulin resistance including impaired glucose tolerance in 6 individuals and type 2 diabetes in 4 [67]. In 39%, hyperinsulinaemia was associated with hypertriglyceridaemia. The frequency of hyperinsulinaemia increased with time from transplantation and abdominal obesity but not overweight was common.

Treatment and Prevention of the Metabolic Syndrome in Survivors of the Treatment of Childhood Cancer

In young adult life [78], weight gain and obesity are linked to hypertension and increased risk of coronary artery disease, and obesity accounts for more than half of the variance in insulin sensitivity in the general population. Elevated total cholesterol concentrations are linked to the risk of cardiovascular disease and reducing cholesterol concentrations in younger people has a greater effect in reducing cardiovascular risk. These findings underlie the importance of identifying modifiable risk factors for cardiovascular disease in young adult survivors of childhood cancer. At the presentation of childhood leukaemia, less than 2% are obese and excess weight gain in a cohort who underwent cranial irradiation does not seem easily predictable from routinely collected data at diagnosis. Therefore, all children treated for childhood ALL should be considered at risk of excess weight gain and the target of appropriate interventions [86].

Limitations of physical performance, executive function and emotional health are negatively associated with both role performance and self-reported health-related quality of life [87]. This finding is important for those designing rehabilitative programmes designed to increase levels of physical activity as they suggest a multidisciplinary approach including physical trainers, physiotherapists, occupational therapists and psychologists will be required to improve outcomes. To date, there are no studies which have evaluated the effectiveness of interventions which aim to modify lifestyle by promoting physical activity and modifying dietary intake with a view to reducing the risk factors for metabolic disorders in survivors of childhood cancer and research in this area is now required.

Given that many of the markers of the metabolic syndrome seen in survivors of childhood cancer are associated with evidence of growth hormone deficiency and that growth hormone treatment may reverse some of these abnormalities, it has been advocated that growth hormone status and lipids should be screened in those survivors who have received therapy which places them at risk of growth hormone deficiency [77]. However, disappointingly, a trial of 12 months of growth hormone therapy in a small cohort of previously irradiated growth hormone-deficient adult survivors of childhood ALL, whilst producing improvements on body composition, failed to have any beneficial effect on pre-existing hyperleptinaemia, hyperinsulinaemia and impaired insulin sensitivity [88]. These findings are in keeping with some studies of the effect of growth hormone replacement in growth hormone-deficient adults in whom treatment failed to reduce the relatively high rates of the metabolic syndrome [89]. By contrast, another similar but longer term study in 18 patients showed not only improvements in body composition and reductions in leptin concentrations after 2 years of growth hormone therapy but also resolution of many features of the metabolic syndrome in all 6 subjects who had evidence of this disorder prior to growth hormone therapy, despite little effect of growth hormone on lipid concentrations. Furthermore, following treatment, there was an increase in the left ventricular mass index and improvement in cardiac systolic function [90]. These findings suggest that where appropriate, growth hormone replacement in combination with diet and lipid-lowering medication and advice regarding cessation of smoking should be considered to reduce the risks of developing cardiovascular disease, though long-term prospective follow-up studies will be required to evaluate the benefits of these interventions.

The question of which patients and how long they should be followed after treatment of childhood cancer and which symptoms and organ functions should be followed into adulthood is often raised [Edgar et al., pp 159–180]. The increasing evidence that growth hormone deficiency may be responsible for the development of a number of metabolic abnormalities in these patients suggests that those who have received cranial irradiation will require long-term follow-up and treatment with growth hormone where appropriate though further studies will be required to evaluate the benefit of therapy. Some patients treated for certain cancers with regimens which were not thought to represent risk factors for growth hormone deficiency may still be at risk of overweight and metabolic disorders in later life [82]. Some have argued that this large and increasing group such as all those who have received chemotherapy alone for ALL should also be followed up [81]. Linked to the issue of follow-up is the extent to which patients should be counselled regarding their condition and increased risks of future adverse health, including metabolic disorders, without inducing unnecessary anxieties. Of relevance to this issue is evidence from a recent survey [91] which shows that young adult survivors of ALL have very poor knowledge levels by comparison with controls about the symptoms which might suggest the onset of angina or a heart attack, conditions which they are at increased risk of experiencing and early identification of which has implications for improving chances of survival. These findings suggest that effective health education will need to be an important part of the longer term follow-up of these patient into later life.

References

1 Isomaa B, Almgren P, Tuomi T, Forsén B, Lahti K, Nissén M, Taskinen MR, Groop L: Cardiovascular morbidity and mortality associated with the metabolic syndrome. Diabetes Care 2001;24:683–689.

2 Lakka HM, Laaksonen DE, Lakka TA, Niskanen LK, Kumpusalo E, Tuomilehto J, Salonen JT: The metabolic syndrome and total and cardiovascular disease mortality in middle-aged men. JAMA 2002;288:2709–2716.

3 Reaven GM: Role of insulin resistance in human disease. Diabetes 1988;37:1595–1607.

4 Björntorp P: Abdominal obesity and the metabolic syndrome. Ann Med 1992;24:465–468.

5 Mykkänen L, Zaccaro DJ, Wagenknecht LE, Robbins DC, Gabriel M, Haffner SM: Microalbuminuria is associated with insulin resistance in nondiabetic subjects: the insulin resistance atherosclerosis study. Diabetes 1998;47:793–800.

6 Yudkin JS: Abnormalities of coagulation and fibrinolysis in insulin resistance. Evidence for a common antecedent? Diabetes Care 1999;22 (suppl 3):C25–C30.
7 Vignesh JP, Mohan V: Polycystic ovary syndrome: a component of metabolic syndrome? J Postgrad Med 2007;53:128–134.
8 Lemieux I, Pascot A, Couillard C, Lamarche B, Tchernof A, Alméras N, Bergeron J, Gaudet D, Tremblay G, Prud'homme D, Nadeau A, Després JP: Hypertriglyceridemic waist: a marker of the atherogenic metabolic triad (hyperinsulinemia; hyperapolipoprotein B; small, dense LDL) in men? Circulation 2000;102:179–184.
9 Eckel RH, Grundy SM, Zimmet PZ: The metabolic syndrome. Lancet 2005;365:1415–1428.
10 Alberti KG, Zimmet P, Shaw J; IDF Epidemiology Task Force Consensus Group: The metabolic syndrome – a new worldwide definition. Lancet 2005; 366:1059–1062.
11 Tan CE, Ma S, Wai D, Chew SK, Tai ES: Can we apply the National Cholesterol Education Program Adult Treatment Panel definition of the metabolic syndrome to Asians? Diabetes Care 2004; 27:1182–1186.
12 Burke V, Beilin LJ, Simmer K, Oddy WH, Blake KV, Doherty D, Kendall GE, Newnham JP, Landau LI, Stanley FJ: Predictors of body mass index and associations with cardiovascular risk factors in Australian children: a prospective cohort study. Int J Obes (Lond) 2005;29:15–23.
13 Ford ES, Giles WH, Dietz WH: Prevalence of the metabolic syndrome among US adults: findings from the third National Health and Nutrition Examination Survey. JAMA 2002;287:356–359.
14 Zimmet P, Alberti G, Kaufman F, Tajima N, Silink M, Arslanian S, Wong G, Bennett P, Shaw J, Caprio S; International Diabetes Federation Task Force on Epidemiology and Prevention of Diabetes: The metabolic syndrome in children and adolescents. Lancet 2007;369:2059–2061.
15 Reinehr T, de Sousa G, Toschke AM, Andler W: Comparison of metabolic syndrome prevalence using eight different definitions: a critical approach. Arch Dis Child 2007;92:1067–1072.
16 Gluckman PD: Evolving a definition of disease. Arch Dis Child 2007;92:1053–1054.
17 Alberti KGMM, Zimmet PZ: Definition, diagnosis and classification of diabetes mellitus and its complications. Part 1: diagnosis and classification of diabetes mellitus provisional report of a WHO consultation. Diabet Med 1998;15:539–555.
18 Lindström J, Louheranta A, Mannelin M, Rastas M, Salminen V, Eriksson J, Uusitupa M, Tuomilehto J; Finnish Diabetes Prevention Study Group: The Finnish Diabetes Prevention Study (DPS): lifestyle intervention and 3-year results on diet and physical activity. Diabetes Care 2003; 26:3230–3236.
19 Bo S, Ciccone G, Baldi C, Benini L, Dusio F, Forastiere G, Lucia C, Nuti C, Durazzo M, Cassader M, Gentile L, Pagano G: Effectiveness of a lifestyle intervention on metabolic syndrome. A randomized controlled trial. J Gen Intern Med 2007; 22:1695–1703.
20 Gurney JG, Ness KK, Sibley SD, O'Leary M, Dengel DR, Lee JM, Youngren NM, Glasser SP, Baker KS: Metabolic syndrome and growth hormone deficiency in adult survivors of childhood acute lymphoblastic leukemia. Cancer 2006;107:1303–1312.
21 Lustig RH, Post SR, Srivannaboon K, Rose SR, Danish RK, Burghen GA, Xiong X, Wu S, Merchant TE: Risk factors for the development of obesity in children surviving brain tumors. J Clin Endocrinol Metab 2003;88:611–616.
22 Warner JT, Evans WD, Webb DK, Gregory JW: Body composition of long-term survivors of acute lymphoblastic leukaemia. Med Pediatr Oncol 2002;38:165–172.
23 Reilly JJ, Ventham JC, Newell J, Aitchison T, Wallace WH, Gibson BE: Risk factors for excess weight gain in children treated for acute lymphoblastic leukaemia. Int J Obes Relat Metab Disord 2000 ;24:1537–1541.
24 Sklar CA, Mertens AC, Walter A, Mitchell D, Nesbit ME, O'Leary M, Hutchinson R, Meadows AT, Robison LL: Changes in body mass index and prevalence of overweight in survivors of childhood acute lymphoblastic leukemia: role of cranial irradiation. Med Pediatr Oncol 2000;35: 91–95.
25 Oeffinger KC, Mertens AC, Sklar CA, Yasui Y, Fears T, Stovall M, Vik TA, Inskip PD, Robison LL; Childhood Cancer Survivor Study: Obesity in adult survivors of childhood acute lymphoblastic leukemia: a report from the Childhood Cancer Survivor Study. J Clin Oncol 2003;21:1359–1365.
26 Ross JA, Oeffinger KC, Davies SM, Mertens AC, Langer EK, Kiffmeyer WR, Sklar CA, Stovall M, Yasui Y, Robison LL: Genetic variation in the leptin receptor gene and obesity in survivors of childhood acute lymphoblastic leukemia: a report from the Childhood Cancer Survivor Study. J Clin Oncol 2004;22:3558–3562.

27 Davies JH, Evans BA, Jones E, Evans WD, Jenney ME, Gregory JW: Osteopenia, excess adiposity and hyperleptinaemia during 2 years of treatment for childhood acute lymphoblastic leukaemia without cranial irradiation. Clin Endocrinol (Oxf) 2004;60:358–365.
28 Grenier MA, Lipshultz SE: Epidemiology of anthracycline cardiotoxicity in children and adults. Semin Oncol 1998;25(suppl 10):72–85.
29 Adams MJ, Hardenbergh PH, Constine LS, Lipshultz SE: Radiation-associated cardiovascular disease. Crit Rev Oncol Hematol 2003;45:55–75.
30 Mertens AC, Yasui Y, Liu Y, Stovall M, Hutchinson R, Ginsberg J, Sklar C, Robison LL; Childhood Cancer Survivor Study: Pulmonary complications in survivors of childhood and adolescent cancer. A report from the Childhood Cancer Survivor Study. Cancer 2002;95:2431–2441.
31 Warner JT, Bell W, Webb DK, Gregory JW: Daily energy expenditure and physical activity in survivors of childhood malignancy. Pediatr Res 1998;43:607–613.
32 Zee P, Chen CH: Prevalence of obesity in children after therapy for acute lymphoblastic leukemia. Am J Pediatr Hematol Oncol 1986;8:294–299.
33 Didi M, Didcock E, Davies HA, Ogilvy-Stuart AL, Wales JK, Shalet SM: High incidence of obesity in young adults after treatment of acute lymphoblastic leukemia in childhood. J Pediatr 1995;127:63–67.
34 Meacham LR, Gurney JG, Mertens AC, Ness KK, Sklar CA, Robison LL, Oeffinger KC: Body mass index in long-term adult survivors of childhood cancer: a report of the Childhood Cancer Survivor Study. Cancer 2005;103:1730–1739.
35 Nathan PC, Jovcevska V, Ness KK, Mammone D'Agostino N, Staneland P, Urbach SL, Barron M, Barrera M, Greenberg ML: The prevalence of overweight and obesity in pediatric survivors of cancer. J Pediatr 2006;149:518–525.
36 Brouwer CA, Gietema JA, Kamps WA, de Vries EG, Postma A: Changes in body composition after childhood cancer treatment: impact on future health status – a review. Crit Rev Oncol Hematol 2007;63:32–46.
37 Warner JT, Cowan FJ, Dunstan FD, Gregory JW: The validity of body mass index for the assessment of adiposity in children with disease states. Ann Hum Biol 1997;24:209–215.
38 Nysom K, Holm K, Michaelsen KF, Hertz H, Müller J, Mølgaard C: Degree of fatness after treatment for acute lymphoblastic leukemia in childhood. J Clin Endocrinol Metab 1999;84: 4591–4596.
39 Sorva R: Children with craniopharyngioma. Early growth failure and rapid postoperative weight gain. Acta Paediatr Scand 1988;77:587–592.
40 Sklar CA: Craniopharyngioma: endocrine sequelae of treatment. Pediatr Neurosurg 1994;21 (suppl 1):120–123.
41 de Vile CJ, Grant DB, Hayward RD, Kendall BE, Neville BG, Stanhope R: Obesity in childhood craniopharyngioma: relation to post-operative hypothalamic damage shown by magnetic resonance imaging. J Clin Endocrinol Metab 1996; 81:2734–2737.
42 Gurney JG, Ness KK, Stovall M, Wolden S, Punyko JA, Neglia JP, Mertens AC, Packer RJ, Robison LL, Sklar CA: Final height and body mass index among adult survivors of childhood brain cancer: childhood cancer survivor study. J Clin Endocrinol Metab 2003;88:4731–4739.
43 Florin TA, Fryer GE, Miyoshi T, Weitzman M, Mertens AC, Hudson MM, Sklar CA, Emmons K, Hinkle A, Whitton J, Stovall M, Robison LL, Oeffinger KC: Physical inactivity in adult survivors of childhood acute lymphoblastic leukemia: a report from the childhood cancer survivor study. Cancer Epidemiol Biomarkers Prev 2007;16:1356–1363.
44 Ness KK, Mertens AC, Hudson MM, Wall MM, Leisenring WM, Oeffinger KC, Sklar CA, Robison LL, Gurney JG: Limitations on physical performance and daily activities among long-term survivors of childhood cancer. Ann Intern Med 2005;143:639–647.
45 Reilly JJ, Blacklock CJ, Dale E, Donaldson M, Gibson BE: Resting metabolic rate and obesity in childhood acute lymphoblastic leukaemia. Int J Obes Relat Metab Disord 1996;20:1130–1132.
46 Warner JT, Bell W, Webb DK, Gregory JW: Relationship between cardiopulmonary response to exercise and adiposity in survivors of childhood malignancy. Arch Dis Child 1997;76:298–303.
47 van Brussel M, Takken T, Lucia A, van der Net J, Helders PJ: Is physical fitness decreased in survivors of childhood leukemia? A systematic review. Leukemia 2005;19:13–17.
48 Gocha Marchese V, Chiarello LA, Lange BJ: Strength and functional mobility in children with acute lymphoblastic leukemia. Med Pediatr Oncol 2003;40:230–232.

49 Hovi L, Era P, Rautonen J, Siimes MA: Impaired muscle strength in female adolescents and young adults surviving leukemia in childhood. Cancer 1993;72:276–281.

50 Ness KK, Baker KS, Dengel DR, Youngren N, Sibley S, Mertens AC, Gurney JG: Body composition, muscle strength deficits and mobility limitations in adult survivors of childhood acute lymphoblastic leukemia. Pediatr Blood Cancer 2007;49:975–981.

51 Talvensaari KK, Jämsen A, Vanharanta H, Lanning M: Decreased isokinetic trunk muscle strength and performance in long-term survivors of childhood malignancies: correlation with hormonal defects. Arch Phys Med Rehabil 1995; 76:983–988.

52 Griggs RC, Kingston W, Jozefowicz RF, Herr BE, Forbes G, Halliday D: Effect of testosterone on muscle mass and muscle protein synthesis. J Appl Physiol 1989;66:498–503.

53 Lipshultz SE, Colan SD, Gelber RD, Perez-Atayde AR, Sallan SE, Sanders SP: Late cardiac effects of doxorubicin therapy for acute lymphoblastic leukemia in childhood. N Engl J Med 1991;324:808–815.

54 Lipshultz SE, Lipsitz SR, Sallan SE, Dalton VM, Mone SM, Gelber RD, Colan SD: Chronic progressive cardiac dysfunction years after doxorubicin therapy for childhood acute lymphoblastic leukemia. J Clin Oncol 2005;23:2629–2636.

55 Quigley C, Cowell C, Jimenez M, Burger H, Kirk J, Bergin M, Stevens M, Simpson J, Silink M: Normal or early development of puberty despite gonadal damage in children treated for acute lymphoblastic leukemia. N Engl J Med 1989;321:143–151.

56 Oberfield SE, Soranno D, Nirenberg A, Heller G, Allen JC, David R, Levine LS, Sklar CA: Age at onset of puberty following high-dose central nervous system radiation therapy. Arch Pediatr Adolesc Med 1996;150:589–592.

57 Sklar C, Mertens A, Walter A, Mitchell D, Nesbit M, O'Leary M, Hutchinson R, Meadows A, Robison L: Final height after treatment for childhood acute lymphoblastic leukemia: comparison of no cranial irradiation with 1800 and 2400 centigrays of cranial irradiation. J Pediatr 1993;123:59–64.

58 Darzy KH, Pezzoli SS, Thorner MO, Shalet SM: The dynamics of growth hormone (GH) secretion in adult cancer survivors with severe GH deficiency acquired after brain irradiation in childhood for nonpituitary brain tumors: evidence for preserved pulsatility and diurnal variation with increased secretory disorderliness. J Clin Endocrinol Metab 2005;90:2794–2803.

59 Salomon F, Cuneo RC, Hesp R, Sönksen PH: The effects of treatment with recombinant human growth hormone on body composition and metabolism in adults with growth hormone deficiency. N Engl J Med 1989;321:1797–1803.

60 Carroll PV, Christ ER, Bengtsson BA, Carlsson L, Christiansen JS, Clemmons D, Hintz R, Ho K, Laron Z, Sizonenko P, Sönksen PH, Tanaka T, Thorne M: Growth hormone deficiency in adulthood and the effects of growth hormone replacement: a review. Growth Hormone Research Society Scientific Committee. J Clin Endocrinol Metab 1998;83:382–395.

61 Brennan BM, Rahim A, Mackie EM, Eden OB, Shalet SM: Growth hormone status in adults treated for acute lymphoblastic leukaemia in childhood. Clin Endocrinol (Oxf) 1998;48:777–783.

62 Talvensaari KK, Lanning M, Tapanainen P, Knip M. Long-term survivors of childhood cancer have an increased risk of manifesting the metabolic syndrome. J Clin Endocrinol Metab 1996;81: 3051–3055.

63 Adan L, Trivin C, Sainte-Rose C, Zucker JM, Hartmann O, Brauner R: GH deficiency caused by cranial irradiation during childhood: factors and markers in young adults. J Clin Endocrinol Metab 2001;86:5245–5251.

64 Màrky I, Mellander L, Lannering B, Albertsson-Wikland K: A longitudinal study of growth and growth hormone secretion in children during treatment for acute lymphoblastic leukemia. Med Pediatr Oncol 1991;19:258–264.

65 Rosén T, Bengtsson BA: Premature mortality due to cardiovascular disease in hypopituitarism. Lancet 1990;336:285–288.

66 Bülow B, Hagmar L, Mikoczy Z, Nordström CH, Erfurth EM: Increased cerebrovascular mortality in patients with hypopituitarism. Clin Endocrinol (Oxf) 1997;46:75–81.

67 Taskinen M, Saarinen-Pihkala UM, Hovi L, Lipsanen-Nyman M: Impaired glucose tolerance and dyslipidaemia as late effects after bone-marrow transplantation in childhood. Lancet 2000;356: 993–997.

68 Neville KA, Cohn RJ, Steinbeck KS, Johnston K, Walker JL: Hyperinsulinemia, impaired glucose tolerance, and diabetes mellitus in survivors of childhood cancer: prevalence and risk factors. J Clin Endocrinol Metab 2006;91:4401–4407.

69 Van Dongen-Melman JE, Hokken-Koelega AC, Hählen K, De Groot A, Tromp CG, Egeler RM: Obesity after successful treatment of acute lymphoblastic leukemia in childhood. Pediatr Res 1995;38:86–90.

70 Brennan BM, Rahim A, Blum WF, Adams JA, Eden OB, Shalet SM: Hyperleptinaemia in young adults following cranial irradiation in childhood: growth hormone deficiency or leptin insensitivity? Clin Endocrinol (Oxf) 1999;50:163–169.

71 Birkebaek NH, Fisker S, Clausen N, Tuovinen V, Sindet-Pedersen S, Christiansen JS: Growth and endocrinological disorders up to 21 years after treatment for acute lymphoblastic leukemia in childhood. Med Pediatr Oncol 1998;30:351–356.

72 Zhang Y, Proenca R, Maffei M, Barone M, Leopold L, Friedman JM: Positional cloning of the mouse obese gene and its human homologue. Nature 1994;372:425–432.

73 Friedman JM, Halaas JL: Leptin and the regulation of body weight in mammals. Nature 1998; 395:763–770.

74 Hawkins MM, Kingston JE, Kinnier Wilson LM: Late deaths after treatment for childhood cancer. Arch Dis Child 1990;65:1356–1363.

75 Nicholson HS, Fears TR, Byrne J: Death during adulthood in survivors of childhood and adolescent cancer. Cancer 1994;73:3094–3102.

76 Talvensaari K, Knip M: Childhood cancer and later development of the metabolic syndrome. Ann Med 1997;29:353–355.

77 Heikens J, Ubbink MC, van der Pal HP, Bakker PJ, Fliers E, Smilde TJ, Kastelein JJ, Trip MD: Long term survivors of childhood brain cancer have an increased risk for cardiovascular disease. Cancer 2000;88:2116–2121.

78 Oeffinger KC, Buchanan GR, Eshelman DA, Denke MA, Andrews TC, Germak JA, Tomlinson GE, Snell LE, Foster BM: Cardiovascular risk factors in young adult survivors of childhood acute lymphoblastic leukemia. J Pediatr Hematol Oncol 2001;23:424–430.

79 Janiszewski PM, Oeffinger KC, Church TS, Dunn AL, Eshelman DA, Victor RG, Brooks S, Turoff AJ, Sinclair E, Murray JC, Bashore L, Ross R: Abdominal obesity, liver fat, and muscle composition in survivors of childhood acute lymphoblastic leukemia. J Clin Endocrinol Metab 2007; 92:3816–3821.

80 Link K, Moëll C, Garwicz S, Cavallin-Ståhl E, Björk J, Thilén U, Ahrén B, Erfurth EM: Growth hormone deficiency predicts cardiovascular risk in young adults treated for acute lymphoblastic leukemia in childhood. J Clin Endocrinol Metab 2004;89:5003–5012.

81 Jarfelt M, Lannering B, Bosaeus I, Johannsson G, Bjarnason R: Body composition in young adult survivors of childhood acute lymphoblastic leukaemia. Eur J Endocrinol 2005;153:81–89.

82 Trimis G, Moschovi M, Papassotiriou I, Chrousos G, Tzortzatou-Stathopoulou F: Early indicators of dysmetabolic syndrome in young survivors of acute lymphoblastic leukemia in childhood as a target for preventing disease. J Pediatr Hematol Oncol 2007;29:309–314.

83 Dengel DR, Ness KK, Glasser SP, Williamson EB, Baker KS, Gurney JG: Endothelial function in young adult survivors of childhood acute lymphoblastic leukemia. J Pediatr Hematol Oncol 2008;30:20–25.

84 Oeffinger KC: Are survivors of acute lymphoblastic leukemia (ALL) at increased risk of cardiovascular disease? Pediatr Blood Cancer 2008; 50(suppl):462–467.

85 Baker KS, Ness KK, Steinberger J, Carter A, Francisco L, Burns LJ, Sklar C, Forman S, Weisdorf D, Gurney JG, Bhatia S: Diabetes, hypertension, and cardiovascular events in survivors of hematopoietic cell transplantation: a report from the bone marrow transplantation survivor study. Blood 2007;109:1765–1772.

86 Reilly JJ, Ventham JC, Newell J, Aitchison T, Wallace WH, Gibson BE: Risk factors for excess weight gain in children treated for acute lymphoblastic leukaemia. Int J Obes Relat Metab Disord 2000;24:1537–1541.

87 Ness KK, Gurney JG, Zeltzer LK, Leisenring W, Mulrooney DA, Nathan PC, Robison LL, Mertens AC: The impact of limitations in physical, executive, and emotional function on health-related quality of life among adult survivors of childhood cancer: a report from the Childhood Cancer Survivor Study. Arch Phys Med Rehabil 2008;89:128–136.

88 Bülow B, Link K, Ahrén B, Nilsson AS, Erfurth EM: Survivors of childhood acute lymphoblastic leukaemia, with radiation-induced GH deficiency, exhibit hyperleptinaemia and impaired insulin sensitivity, unaffected by 12 months of GH treatment. Clin Endocrinol (Oxf) 2004;61: 683–691.

89 van der Klaauw AA, Biermasz NR, Feskens EJ, Bos MB, Smit JW, Roelfsema F, Corssmit EP, Pijl H, Romijn JA, Pereira AM: The prevalence of the metabolic syndrome is increased in patients with GH deficiency, irrespective of long-term substitution with recombinant human GH. Eur J Endocrinol 2007;156:455–462.

90 Follin C, Thilén U, Ahrén B, Erfurth EM: Improvement in cardiac systolic function and reduced prevalence of metabolic syndrome after two years of growth hormone (GH) treatment in GH-deficient adult survivors of childhood-onset acute lymphoblastic leukemia. J Clin Endocrinol Metab 2006;91:1872–1875.

91 Gurney JG, Donohue JE, Ness KK, O'Leary M, Glasser SP, Baker KS: Health knowledge about symptoms of heart attack and stroke in adult survivors of childhood acute lymphoblastic leukemia. Ann Epidemiol 2007;17:778–781.

Prof. John W. Gregory
Professor in Paediatric Endocrinology
Department of Child Health, Wales School of Medicine, Cardiff University
Heath Park
Cardiff CF14 4XN (UK)
Tel. +44 2920 742 274, Fax +44 2920 745 438, E-Mail wchjwg@cardiff.ac.uk

Wallace WHB, Kelnar CJH (eds): Endocrinopathy after Childhood Cancer Treatment.
Endocr Dev. Basel, Karger, 2009, vol 15, pp 77–100

Bone and Bone Turnover

Patricia M. Crofton

Department of Paediatric Biochemistry, Royal Hospital for Sick Children, University of Edinburgh, Edinburgh, UK

Abstract

Children with cancer are exposed to multiple influences that may adversely affect bone health. Some treatments have direct deleterious effects on bone whilst others may have indirect effects mediated through various endocrine abnormalities. Most clinical outcome studies have concentrated on survivors of acute lymphoblastic leukaemia (ALL). There is now good evidence that earlier treatment protocols that included cranial irradiation with doses of 24 Gy or greater may result in growth hormone deficiency and low bone mineral density (BMD) in the lumbar spine and femoral neck. Under current protocols, BMD decreases during intensive chemotherapy and fracture risk increases. Although total body BMD may eventually return to normal after completion of chemotherapy, lumbar spine trabecular BMD may remain low for many years. The implications for long-term fracture risk are unknown. Risk factors for low BMD include high dose methotrexate, higher cumulative doses of glucocorticoids, male gender and low physical activity. BMD outcome in non-ALL childhood cancers has been less well studied but there is evidence that survivors of childhood brain or bone tumours, and survivors of bone marrow transplants for childhood malignancy, all have a high risk of long-term osteopenia. Long-term follow-up is required, with appropriate treatment of any endocrine abnormalities identified.

During childhood, bone growth involves both longitudinal growth and growth in width. Longitudinal growth occurs at the growth plate by endochondral ossification, with progressive creation of new bone at the lower end of the growth plate. This process is governed by a host of endocrine signals, including growth hormone (GH), insulin-like growth factor-1 (IGF-1), thyroid hormone, oestrogen, androgen, glucocorticoids (GCs) and vitamin D. These interact with each other and also with a complex network of paracrine and autocrine factors within the growth plate. Growth in bone width occurs by a modelling process during which osteoblasts deposit new bone on the outer periosteal surface, while osteoclasts simultaneously resorb bone from the inner endocortical surface, resulting in a net

Table 1. Definitions of bone mass parameters

Bone parameter	Abbreviation	Units	Definition
Bone mineral content	BMC	mg/mm or mg/cm	Mass of bone mineral per unit of axial bone length
Bone mineral density	vBMD	g/cm^3	True volumetric bone mineral density measured by QCT within the specified compartment
Areal bone mineral 'density'	aBMD	g/cm^2	Degree of attenuation of a radiation beam by bone, based on a two-dimensional projected image, as measured by DEXA Reflects a combination of physical density and size
Bone mineral apparent density	BMAD	g/cm^3	aBMD corrected for bone size by a variety of mathematical formulae, usually assuming vertebral shape is either a cube or a cylinder May over- or under-correct for bone size. Does not equate to vBMD by QCT

increase in cortical thickness and bone width [1]. Additionally, in both children and adults all bone undergoes continual remodelling. This involves a sequential process of osteoclastic resorption of a small quantity of bone tissue, followed by osteoblastic bone formation during which the cavity is re-filled with new bone. These processes are normally tightly coupled so that net bone balance is close to zero. However, under some circumstances, the activation frequency of bone remodelling units may increase, leading to an overall increase in bone turnover and net bone loss.

Bone strength – and hence fracture risk – is dependent on a combination of its inherent structural composition and its geometry. Bone mineral density (BMD) is sometimes used as a surrogate for fracture risk, but is only one variable contributing to fracture risk. At the present time, true volumetric BMD (vBMD, g/cm^3) can only be measured by quantitative computed tomography (QCT), usually either at the lumbar spine or the distal radius (table 1). However, in clinical practice, BMD is usually measured by dual energy X-ray absorptiometry (DEXA), either whole body or at various skeletal sites. This is not true vBMD but so-called 'areal' BMD (aBMD, g/cm^2) reflecting a combination of physical density and size (table 1). A low aBMD may be caused by either a low vBMD or reduced bone size. To overcome this, a derived variable, called bone mineral apparent density (BMAD), is sometimes calculated from the aBMD; this corrects for bone size using various mathematical formulae which may either over- or under-correct for bone size. It does not equate to true vBMD as measured by QCT.

Because it depends partly on bone size, aBMD varies markedly with age and gender throughout childhood. For this reason, it is often expressed as a z score (standard deviation score), defined as: (measured aBMD – population mean aBMD for healthy children of the same age and gender)/(population aBMD standard deviation).

The overall balance between bone formation and bone resorption contributes to net outcome in terms of BMD. These processes can be assessed by bone histomorphometry but this procedure is rarely performed in children because of the obvious ethical difficulties in carrying out invasive bone biopsies and uncertainties regarding the optimal site. Instead, measurement of biochemical markers of bone formation and resorption may be used to give real time insight into bone dynamics. Bone formation markers include procollagen type I C- or N-terminal propeptide (PICP or PINP, markers of type I collagen synthesis), bone alkaline phosphatase (ALP, produced by the osteoblast) and osteocalcin (also produced by the osteoblast). There are a plethora of bone resorption markers, including deoxypyridinoline, the N-telopeptide of type I collagen (both measured in urine), or the cross-linked telopeptide of type I collagen (ICTP or CrossLaps), measured in plasma. Because all these markers vary markedly during childhood in a pattern reflecting the childhood growth curve, they may also be expressed as z scores in relation to age- and gender-matched normal children.

Children with cancer are exposed to multiple influences that may adversely affect bone health. These include the disease process itself, radiotherapy, chemotherapy, poor nutrition and lack of physical activity. Any combination of these factors may result in osteopenia, failure to attain optimal peak bone mass and predisposition to later osteoporosis.

A number of outcome studies have investigated BMD in survivors of childhood cancer, reflecting the cumulative effects of many years of multiple influences on bone. However, if osteopenia is found, it can be difficult to dissect out the causes. Furthermore, treatment protocols are constantly being refined and improved; retrospective outcome studies can only address the effects of earlier, often heterogeneous protocols, some of which have since become obsolete. To evaluate bone pathology in children treated for cancer and to gain insight into causes and mechanisms, several complementary approaches are required. Each has advantages and potential pitfalls. In clinical practice, fracture risk is the most important outcome but is the most difficult to quantify, requiring an unrealistic sample size and very long follow-up. BMD is the next most relevant outcome measure but is only a surrogate for fracture risk and it may be difficult to interpret aBMD in children whose treatment has resulted in impaired growth, delayed puberty and/or reduced final height, owing to the confounding effects of bone size (see above). Clinical studies employing serial measurements of biochemical markers of bone metabolism and selected hormones may dissect out the dynamic effects of each phase of treatment on whole body bone turnover and give insight into mechanisms but cannot give information on particular bone sites, nor can they definitively separate out individual versus synergistic effects of each component of a multi-drug regimen. Serial histomorphometry in animal models is useful in studying the effects of individual drugs on bone in the intact organism but requires caution in extrapolating to human children. Studies on cultured human bone cells have enabled researchers to tease out the effects of individual drugs and hormones at the cellular level, alone or in combination, but these findings may not be directly applicable to the child treated for cancer. All these approaches are complementary and together have helped to increase our understanding of the causes of osteopenia in survivors of childhood cancer.

Treatments for Childhood Cancer: Effects on Bone

Treatments for childhood cancer may have either direct or indirect effects on bone.

Radiation Damage

Spinal irradiation causes direct, dose-dependent damage to vertebrae, although this may take months or years to become evident. Although spinal irradiation is avoided where possible in most modern treatment protocols, craniospinal irradiation is still used for the treatment of certain cancers, e.g. intracranial space-occupying lesions such as medulloblastoma.

Cranial irradiation may cause decreased longitudinal bone growth and/or inadequate bone mass acquisition mediated mainly by GH deficiency. In some survivors TSH or LH/FSH deficiency may also play a role (see below). Radiation damage occurs mainly at the hypothalamic level and is dose-dependent. GH is the most susceptible of the pituitary hormones and deficiency may occur at doses of 24 Gy or greater when given in conventional daily fractions [2]. GH plays a key role not only in longitudinal bone growth but also in attainment of peak bone mass. Although true vBMD is usually normal in patients with untreated childhood-onset GH deficiency, adult peak bone mass and size are low, leading to decreased bone strength and increased fracture risk [3]. Retrospective outcome studies on survivors of childhood acute lymphoblastic leukaemia (ALL) and/or brain tumours who have been treated with cranial irradiation have demonstrated blunted GH responses to provocative testing, the degree of impairment being related to radiation dose [2, 4, 5]. Survivors also have reduced spontaneous pulsatile GH secretion. Deficiencies in TSH and/or LH/FSH are less frequent after cranial irradiation and tend to occur only after radiation doses around 30–40 Gy. Any deficiency may appear months to years after radiation exposure, necessitating careful follow-up.

Thyroid hormone is a major regulator of normal skeletal development and growth before puberty, with multiple actions on the growth plate. On the other hand, untreated hyperthyroidism may cause accelerated bone loss. Primary hypothyroidism or, less frequently, hyperthyroidism may occur after neck irradiation, such as that used in the treatment of Hodgkin's lymphoma [2].

Sex steroids are required to achieve a normal growth spurt during puberty, when they work synergistically with GH. Additionally, oestrogen is required to maintain bone health in both sexes. In males, oestrogen is formed by aromatisation of testosterone and thus is dependent on adequate testosterone levels. Patients who are deficient in oestrogen or testosterone may have a reduced or absent pubertal growth spurt, reduced bone mass and may eventually develop osteoporosis. Testicular irradiation at doses >24 Gy, such as those used for young males with testicular relapse of ALL, is associated with a high risk of Leydig cell dysfunction, with a consequent requirement for puberty induction and androgen replacement. After exposure to lower radiation doses below 20 Gy, most males go through normal puberty and most produce normal adult levels of testosterone, but LH may be moderately increased in some, indicating compensated Leydig cell dysfunction. In females, abdominal, pelvic or spinal irradiation may cause primary ovarian failure, especially if both ovaries were within the treatment field.

Gonadal Damage: Non-Radiation Causes

Clearly, patients of both sexes in whom both gonads have been removed – most often because of a germ cell tumour – will have oestrogen and/or testosterone deficiency requiring life-long replacement, not only for sexual health but also to maintain bone health.

Most males treated with chemotherapy alone experience normal pubertal development and a normal pubertal growth spurt. However, high doses of some alkylating agents during treatment of childhood cancer may cause subtle damage to Leydig cells. There is evidence that these male survivors may be at risk of reduced BMD of the femoral neck and lumbar spine in adulthood [6].

Ovaries of prepubertal girls are relatively resistant to chemotherapy-induced damage compared with adult ovaries, but nevertheless females who receive high-dose myeloablative therapy with alkylating drugs such as busulphan, melphalan and cyclophosphamide as conditioning treatment before bone marrow transplantation (BMT) have a high risk of developing primary ovarian failure.

Chemotherapy

Glucocorticoids

Glucocorticoids (GCs) are frequently used in the treatment of childhood cancer, either as part of the chemotherapy protocol (for example in ALL) or as an antiemetic. They have many complex and diverse actions on bone, the net result of which is an adverse outcome in terms of longitudinal bone growth and BMD. It is now well established that GCs exert direct actions on the growth plate where they down-regulate GH receptor expression, reduce local production of IGF-1, inhibit chondrocyte proliferation and matrix mineralisation, increase hypertrophic chondrocyte apoptosis and down-regulate vascular endothelial growth factor expression, resulting in impaired endochondral ossification [7]. Removal of GCs allows the resting population of immature chondrocytes to re-enter the chondrogenic pathway, resulting in catch-up growth.

GCs also have a dose-dependent inhibitory effect on osteoblast proliferation and type I collagen synthesis [8]. In animal models, high-dose GC treatment results in decreased BMD, trabecular narrowing, a decrease in histomorphometric variables of bone formation, increased osteoblast apoptosis and decreased serum osteocalcin, with reversal of these effects after weaning off steroids [9]. Bone biopsies taken from patients on long-term GC treatment reveal decreased bone matrix apposition rates, decreased trabecular volume and increased osteoblast apoptosis [8]. Some GC effects may be mediated through decreased IGF-1 synthesis in osteoblasts. In children, as in animal models, GCs suppress markers of collagen formation, with rapid recovery after stopping treatment.

The effects of GCs on osteoclasts and bone degradation are more controversial. However, most evidence indicates that GCs suppress osteoclast function. In animal models, they cause decreased osteoclast production and impaired bone resorption [9] and in children they suppress plasma and urinary markers of bone collagen degradation, with a rebound to supra-physiological levels after weaning off steroids. They also inhibit renal tubular reabsorption of calcium, resulting in hypercalciuria and it has been suggested that secondary hyperparathyroidism may contribute to the osteopenia observed in patients on long-term GC therapy [8].

Methotrexate

Methotrexate has no effect on chondrocyte proliferation or differentiation and no effect on growth in children [7, 10]. However, some children with ALL treated under early protocols using methotrexate as the sole chemotherapeutic agent developed bone pain, osteoporotic fractures and impaired bone healing [10]. In animal models, histomorphometric studies have demonstrated that methotrexate treatment results in osteopenia, markedly reduced trabecular bone volume, low rates of bone formation and mineral apposition, but marked increases in osteoclast number [11]. These adverse histomorphometric effects persist long after cessation of treatment, with no signs of recovery. Methotrexate treatment of cultured human osteoblasts results in a marked dose-dependent reduction in cell numbers but osteoblast phenotypic expression in terms of type I collagen synthesis, ALP or osteocalcin is preserved [12, 13]. These animal and cell culture studies have clinical relevance for current ALL chemotherapy protocols. We have observed that children with ALL who received high dose methotrexate chemotherapy had lower markers of bone formation and higher ICTP (bone resorption) than in those who did not, confirming impaired bone formation and enhanced bone degradation in these children [14].

Ifosfamide

Ifosfamide is an alkylating agent used in several chemotherapy protocols, including osteosarcoma and Ewing's sarcoma protocols. Ifosfamide affects bone indirectly through its nephrotoxic effects resulting in renal phosphate wasting. Risk factors include younger age and higher cumulative doses of ifosfamide [15]. Severe nephrotoxicity may develop progressively and/or persist for several years after completion of treatment, necessitating long-term follow-up of these patients. In a small study of 13 childhood cancer survivors previously treated with chemotherapy protocols that included ifosfamide, mean aBMD at the lumbar spine was low and 3 of 13 children had aBMD z scores of <2.0 [16].

Other Chemotherapeutic Agents

Although less studied than GCs and methotrexate, several other chemotherapeutic agents used in the treatment of childhood cancer have the potential to damage the growth plate or adversely affect bone formation. In rat tibial chondrocyte cultures, the DNA-damaging agents cisplatin, etoposide, carboplatin and actinomycin D all target proliferating chondrocytes, causing irreversible cell loss, whilst the purine anti-metabolites, 6-mercaptopurine and thioguanine, merely slow chondrocyte proliferation [17]. Doxorubicin decreases bone formation in rats, resulting in decreased trabecular bone volume in as little as 5 days [18]. In a series of experiments using human osteoblast cell cultures, vincristine, daunorubicin, cytarabine, etoposide and, to a lesser extent, thioguanine and mercaptopurine were all found to cause a dose-dependent decrease in cell numbers [12]. These decreases were similar to those observed in leukaemic cells when the same agents were used in similar concentrations. Pre-treatment with GCs appears to ameliorate (although not abolish) the cytotoxic effects of many chemotherapeutic agents on both chondrocytes and osteoblasts [12, 19]. This may have relevance for chemotherapy protocols that combine cytotoxic agents with GCs. However, care must be exercised in extrapolating from cell culture experiments to the intact organism, in which many other mineral, endocrine, paracrine and autocrine factors, including growth factors and cytokines, may modulate the effects of cytotoxic drugs on bone.

Clinical Studies

Acute Lymphoblastic Leukaemia

At Diagnosis

At diagnosis, a large proportion of children with ALL have radiographic abnormalities in bone, including lytic lesions, with 10% showing radiographic evidence of fractures [20]. Although some investigators have reported relatively normal lumbar spine aBMD at diagnosis [21, 22], others have reported low aBMD of the lumbar spine [23] or femoral neck [22]. Bone formation markers are low or very low whilst bone resorption markers have been variously reported as very low, low or normal [14, 21, 23, 24]. IGF-1, IGF-binding protein 3 (IGFBP-3) and GH-binding protein (a measure of GH receptor status) are also low at diagnosis, whereas urinary GH is increased [14, 23]. Taken together, the evidence suggests that children with ALL are in a GH-resistant state resulting in markedly reduced bone formation that, depending on timescale, may result in a modest reduction in BMD at diagnosis and increased fracture risk due to the disease process itself.

Effects of Treatment

Chemotherapy protocols for ALL differ from country to country but generally consist of an induction phase, a central nervous system (CNS)-directed therapy phase, followed by a number of blocks of intensive chemotherapy, and finally by a prolonged continuing treatment or maintenance phase. The duration of chemotherapy is 2–3 years and may have a significant impact on growth and bone health. The most intensive chemotherapy is generally given during the first 6 months. Although cranial irradiation was frequently given as CNS-directed therapy in the past, this is now avoided in most cases. On the other hand, there has been a trend towards increasingly intensive chemotherapy in more recent protocols. All regimens include GCs (prednisolone or dexamethasone, given continuously during induction, and as pulse therapy during CNS-directed and maintenance phases) and oral methotrexate. Some also give high dose intravenous methotrexate as CNS-directed therapy. Many other drugs are used in various combinations, depending on the protocal.

It has been reported that up to 40% children may develop fractures during ALL chemotherapy, associated with declining lumbar spine aBMC z scores [21]. One retrospective case-note review compared two consecutive periods when prednisone or dexamethasone were used during post-remission therapy [25]. Overall, the 5-year cumulative incidence of fractures was 28%, dexamethasone being associated with a higher fracture risk than prednisone. However, this was not a randomised controlled trial. In Finnish ALL patients studied at completion of treatment, lumbar spine and femoral neck BMAD were both low (mean z scores –0.8 and –1.0, respectively) [26]. In a prospective study of children treated using Dutch protocols, aBMD of the lumbar spine, already low at diagnosis, remained low throughout treatment with no improvement 1 year after completion of treatment [23]. Total body aBMD was normal at diagnosis but decreased rapidly in the first 6 months when chemotherapy was relatively intense, and showed no improvement at 1-year follow-up. Fracture rate was 6 times higher in ALL patients compared with healthy controls and occurred not only during treatment but also in the first year after completion of treatment. In a similar study conducted in Greece, lumbar spine aBMD z scores were relatively normal at diagnosis but declined considerably in the first 6 months of treatment, then increased to normal at completion of treatment [22]. Femoral neck aBMD z scores were low at diagnosis, decreased further at 6 months, then gradually improved although they remained slightly low at completion of treatment.

Measurement of bone turnover markers is a useful way to assess the dynamic state of bone in real time during chemotherapy and complements BMD measurements which can only be done at intervals of 6 months or more. Two prospective studies have investigated short-term changes in bone markers during induction chemotherapy [14, 24]. Bone formation markers – already low at diagnosis – were suppressed further during induction chemotherapy, accompanied by either an increase [24] or lesser suppression [14] of ICTP (bone resorption marker), presumably resulting in negative bone balance. IGF-1 and IGFBP-3 returned to normal from the low levels observed at diagnosis, and the initial high urinary GH decreased, consistent with a restoration of GH sensitivity as patients entered remission [14]. The effects of induction chemotherapy on bone turnover markers were independent of circulating IGF-1 and IGFBP-3, suggesting a direct effect at the target tissue level. During this period, children also demonstrated decreased height and negative lower leg growth, implying a severe direct adverse effect on the growth plate, in keeping with in vitro experiments. Markers of bone formation and resorption were further suppressed during a 1-week period of intensified chemotherapy [14]. Then, after weaning off steroids, there was a dramatic rebound increase in markers of bone formation and resorption consistent with a resumption of osteoblast proliferation and enhanced bone turnover. This was again independent of circulating IGF-1 and IGFBP-3, which showed little change over this period. The marked increase in bone turnover preceded resumption of lower leg growth.

During the maintenance phase of chemotherapy in year 2, markers of bone collagen formation and resorption, height z scores and growth were all similar to healthy children [27]. However, bone ALP remained low suggesting a defect in osteoblast function, and did not return to normal until after chemotherapy finished. The main culprit is likely to have been methotrexate given weekly throughout maintenance chemotherapy. Prednisolone and vincristine are administered less frequently, and cell culture experiments suggest that co-administration of prednisolone may protect osteoblasts from the cytotoxic effects of vincristine [12].

Long-Term Outcome Studies

Although markers of bone turnover return to normal after completion of treatment and remain normal thereafter [27–30], there have been concerns that the combined effects of the underlying disease process, cranial irradiation in older protocols, increasingly intensive chemotherapy and prolonged exposure to GC and methotrexate during maintenance chemotherapy may adversely affect bone mineral acquisition in puberty, attainment of peak bone mass and future bone health.

A number of cross-sectional studies have investigated BMD outcome after treatment of childhood ALL (table 2). These vary in terms of age at the time of the follow-up study, length of follow-up and whether or not patients had received cranial irradiation as part of their treatment. Most studies confirm that cranial irradiation, as used in older protocols, is a risk factor for low BMD, especially in the lumbar spine [33–35, 38], although two were not able to demonstrate this [36, 37]. In one study [37], this was probably because patients received only 18 Gy which may be below the radiation dose that affects hypothalamic-pituitary function. Kaste et al. [33] found that survivors treated with 24 Gy had lower lumbar spine trabecular vBMD than those who had received 18 Gy or no radiation; there was no difference in BMD between those who had received 18 Gy and those who had received no radiation. The low DEXA lumbar spine aBMDs observed in irradiated patients were not solely due to reduced bone size because trabecular vBMD by QCT was also low [28, 33, 34].

Only a few studies have linked GH status after cranial irradiation to BMD outcome. Nussey et al. [32] reported that 62% of survivors who had received cranial irradiation were GH-deficient (GHD) as diagnosed on clinical criteria alone, although only half of these were on GH treatment. Survivors with untreated GHD had low aBMD in the lumbar spine and femoral neck, whereas those without GHD or who had GH-treated GHD had normal aBMD. There was no attempt to correct aBMD for bone size which may have been smaller in untreated GHD survivors. In keeping with a link between GH status and BMD outcome, Hoorweg-Nijman et al. [29] found low IGF-1 and IGFBP-3 levels in young adult survivors, nearly all of whom had received cranial irradiation, together with low aBMD in the lumbar spine and femoral neck. Brennan et al. [28] formally assessed GH status in young adult survivors, all of whom had received cranial irradiation, using two provocative tests of GH secretion. They found that aBMD was low both in the lumbar spine and femoral neck, and lumbar spine trabecular vBMD was also low, regardless of GH status. It may be that the provocative tests did not reflect the more subtle reductions in spontaneous pulsatile GH secretion that have been described after cranial irradiation [4, 5]. However, Jarfelt et al. [36] also found no relationship between low BMD and GH status, assessed by a 24-hour spontaneous GH profile.

As chemotherapy regimens have intensified over time, there has been concern that chemotherapy alone may adversely affect bone mass accretion during childhood and hence peak bone mass in adult survivors. Studies of BMD outcome in ALL survivors who received only chemotherapy (no radiation) have necessarily been on subjects who were younger at the time of BMD evaluation, with shorter follow-up, compared with studies of survivors who followed earlier protocols involving cranial irradiation and less intensive chemotherapy (table 2). Some studies have demonstrated no adverse effect of chemotherapy on total body or lumbar spine aBMD [39–41]. By contrast, lumbar spine trabecular vBMD was found to be low in ALL survivors treated with chemotherapy alone [42], as was distal radial trabecular vBMD [41], suggesting a possible defect in trabecular bone. Chemotherapy risk factors for low BMD outcome have been identified as high dose methotrexate [37, 40] and/or higher dose GCs [36, 37]. One study compared long-term BMD outcome in patients treated with a protocol containing prednisolone (of whom 40% also received cranial irradiation) and a protocol containing dexamethasone (no cranial irradiation) [43]. No difference in total body or lumbar spine BMD or BMAD outcome between the two protocols was observed.

Only two studies have undertaken serial measurements of BMD in ALL survivors who received chemotherapy alone. Marinovic et al. [30] studied ALL survivors initially between 0 and 3 years after completion of chemotherapy, then again 1 year later. Total body aBMD was slightly lower than controls at first evaluation but not at follow-up. Lumbar spine aBMD was low compared with controls at both evaluations. By the end of the study, the fracture rate in ALL survivors over the previous 5 years was twice that in controls, including some fractures occurring after completion of treatment. Kaste et al. [42] studied children over a longer period of follow-up with two lumbar spine QCT measurements 2–5 years apart, at mean follow-up times of 11 and 16 years after diagnosis respectively. Lumbar spine trabecular vBMD was low at first evaluation (table 2), increased slightly at second evaluation but remained low in relation to population norms. There is therefore evidence of slight improvement with time after completion of chemotherapy but

Table 2. BMD outcome after ALL in childhood

Country	n	Cranial irradiation %	Age at study years	Length of follow-up years	aBMD by DEXA (z score)			LS trabecular vBMD by QCT (z score)	Reference
					total body	lumbar spine	femoral neck		
UK	31	100[a]	23 (18–33)	18[b] (7–29)	–	–0.7 (–2.1 to +1.0)	–0.4 (–1.4 to +1.7)	–1.3 (–3.5 to +1.0)	28
UK	35	100	12	7[c] (3–13)	normal vs. controls	low vs. controls	low vs. controls	–	31
Netherlands	24	92	25 (20–35)	(5–22)	–	–1.1 (–4.2 to +0.5)	–1.1 (–3.6 to +1.0)	–	29
UK	43	91[a]	~21	(10–23)	–	untreated GHD: low non-GHD: normal	untreated GHD: low non-GHD: normal	–	32
USA	141	70	16 (10–30)	(9–15)[c]	–	–	–	–0.8 (low in 21%)	33
USA	42	69	12	4[b] (0.5–11)	–	–	–	non-CI: +0.2 CI: –0.9	34
Finland	29	69	17 (12–30)	8[b] (2–20)	–	low vs. controls	low vs. controls	–	35
Sweden	35	54	(20–32)	20[b]	+0.4 (–1.1 to +2.4)	–0.4 (–2.2 to +2.6) osteopenia in 23%	–0.1 (–2.2 to +2.2) osteopenia in 11%	–	36
Canada	106	50	16 (8–31)	(2–12)[b]	–	+0.02 (–2.9 to +5.2) z score <–1 in 22%	low in 21%	–	37
Denmark	95	41	16 (6–34)	11[c] (3–23)	–0.4 (–3.2 to –2.4)	–0.6 (–3.0 to +1.8)	–	–	38
Netherlands	23	none	(12–25)	10[b] (8–11)	+0.2 (–1.8 to +2.6)	+0.3 (–1.5 to +2.5)	–	–	39

Table 2. (Continued)

Country	n	Cranial irradiation %	Age at study years	Length of follow-up years	aBMD by DEXA (z score)			LS trabecular vBMD by QCT (z score)	Reference
					total body	lumbar spine	femoral neck		
UK	28	none	(6–15)	5^{b}	normal vs. controls	normal vs. controls	–	–	40
UK	53	none	11 (6–17)	$>1^{b}$	normal vs. controls	normal vs. controls	–	–	41
France	37	none	8 (4–20)	2 (0.1–3)	slightly low vs. controls	low vs. controls	–	–	30
USA	57	none	15 (10–31)	12^{c}	–	–	–	–0.6 (–3.2 to +3.2)	42

LS = Lumbar spine; CI = cranial irradiation; GHD = growth hormone deficiency. Data are expressed as the mean or median (range), where this information is provided.
[a] Spinal irradiation (24 Gy) or total body irradiation/BMT also given in a few subjects.
[b] From completion of treatment.
[c] From diagnosis.

nevertheless BMD z scores may remain low for many years after completion of chemotherapy, especially in the lumbar spine.

Male gender was identified by several studies as a risk factor for low BMD outcome, not only among those treated with cranial irradiation but also in those who received only chemotherapy [30, 33, 35, 40]. It is possible that this could be attributable to greater sensitivity to cytotoxic gonadal damage and/or GCs in males, but this explanation remains speculative. Poor exercise tolerance and/or physical activity were also associated with a poorer BMD outcome in the lumbar spine or femoral neck [31, 36, 40]. Markers of bone turnover were correlated to physical performance in one study and the authors concluded that physical fitness was an important factor in developing and preserving normal BMD after childhood ALL [36].

Solid Tumours

There have been fewer studies of BMD and bone turnover in children with solid tumours compared with children treated for ALL.

At Diagnosis

BMAD at the lumbar spine and femoral neck appears to be normal in patients with solid tumours at diagnosis [44]. In a separate study of children with a variety of solid tumours, IGF-1 and bone formation markers were low at diagnosis – although not as low as in children with ALL – whilst the bone resorption marker, ICTP, was normal [45]. This pattern is consistent with an imbalance between bone formation and resorption, probably related to low IGF-1.

Effects of Treatment

Children with solid tumours may receive a wide variety of chemotherapy and radiotherapy protocols. In general, unlike in ALL patients, chemotherapy is given in short intensive courses interspersed with treatment-free intervals, and is often of shorter overall duration. This may potentially allow recovery of bone function between treatment courses and have a lesser impact on overall bone health than the very prolonged ALL treatment schedules. Nevertheless, several drugs used in the treatment of solid tumours have been shown to have adverse actions on cultured chondrocytes (cisplatin, carboplatin, etoposide, actinomycin D), cultured osteoblasts (vincristine, etoposide, daunorubicin) or renal tubules (ifosfamide) [7, 12, 15]. Furthermore, GCs are often given as an anti-emetic during treatment. These may ameliorate the adverse effects of some other agents on chondrocytes and osteoblasts [7, 12] but may have their own deleterious effects on bone.

During chemotherapy (no radiation) of children with a mixture of non-ALL cancers, a decrease in height z score was reported, with recovery shortly after completing treatment [45]. Lower leg length growth velocity was low throughout treatment but also increased after stopping treatment. Samples collected immediately before each treatment course showed a gradual increase in IGF-1 and PICP (bone formation marker), from low levels at diagnosis to normal within the first few cycles. However, although bone ALP also gradually increased, z scores remained low, suggesting an adverse effect on osteoblast function that persisted throughout treatment. ICTP (bone resorption) increased to levels higher than controls over the same period, suggesting a moderate excess of bone collagen degradation over synthesis throughout treatment. Both collagen markers showed a cyclical pattern, decreasing markedly after each course of intensive chemotherapy but recovering between courses. This pattern was attributed to the high dose dexamethasone administered as an anti-emetic in conjunction with each chemotherapy course, causing marked suppression of collagen turnover. Some children with lymphoma did not receive dexamethasone, but did receive prednisolone as part of their chemotherapy: these children had an identical cyclical pattern in their collagen markers.

In a prospective Finnish study on children with cancer, Arikoski et al. [44] reported decreases in BMAD in the lumbar spine and femoral neck over the first 6 months of treatment in patients with solid tumours, similar to those they observed in ALL patients in the same study. At completion of treatment, children with solid tumours had low femoral neck BMAD (mean z score –0.8) but normal lumbar spine BMAD [26]. This contrasts with the lower BMAD found at both sites in ALL patients in the same study, suggesting that treatment of solid tumours has a somewhat less deleterious effect than ALL protocols.

Long-Term Outcome Studies

There have been few long-term BMD outcome studies in patients with solid tumours. Warner et al. [31] studied 20 long-term survivors of various non-ALL childhood cancers at a median age of 11 years, 1.5–12 years after completion of treatment. In the non-ALL cancer survivors, BMC was slightly lower at the lumbar spine and femoral neck compared with controls but not as low as in ALL survivors in the same study.

Odame et al. [46] studied BMD outcome in 25 survivors of childhood brain tumours, of whom half had received cranial or craniospinal irradiation at doses generally exceeding 45 Gy. Age at time of study was 5–23 (median 15) years and follow-up from completion of treatment was 2–16 years. Three patients had GH deficiency, all treated with GH. Whole body and lumbar spine aBMD z scores were relatively normal in the non-irradiated group but much lower in the irradiated group (–1.9 and –1.6, respectively). 67% of the irradiated group had osteopenia (defined as a lumbar spine aBMD z score below –1.0) and 42% had osteoporosis (defined as a whole body aBMD z score <2.5). Three patients (all irradiated) had a history of fractures following completion of therapy. Quality of life assessments demonstrated that pain was more severe and ambulation more restricted in those with low aBMD. There is therefore a strong link between cranial irradiation at doses of >45 Gy and markedly low BMD with associated morbidity.

Two studies have investigated BMD outcome in survivors of bone tumours in childhood or adolescence. The first investigated BMD outcome over a relatively short follow-up period (3–6 years) in 36 adolescent survivors of childhood bone tumours [47]. Height and weight of survivors were similar to the population mean, all had normal full puberty and all had completed linear growth. Lumbar spine aBMD z scores were equally low in osteosarcoma and Ewings sarcoma survivors (mean –0.6), with males having lower z scores (–0.9) than females (–0.2). This increased susceptibility to lower BMD z scores in males is similar to that seen in survivors of childhood ALL and may reflect blunted bone mass accretion at puberty. The second study reported long-term BMD outcome in 48 adults (mean age at time of study 31 years, mean follow-up 16 years) who had been treated during childhood or adolescence for osteosarcoma [48]. All had received chemotherapy using protocols that included high-dose methotrexate, doxorubicin and cyclophosphamide and, additionally in different combinations, bleomycin, dactinomycin, vincristine, cisplatin and ifosfamide. 21% of adult survivors had osteoporosis according to World Health Organisation guidelines, 44% had osteopenia and only 35% had normal BMD.

Bone Marrow Transplant

BMT may be used to treat patients with cancer following relapse after first-line treatment has failed. Various myeloablative conditioning regimens may be employed, comprising either high-dose chemotherapy or total body irradiation or both. These may affect bone directly or indirectly. The pathogenesis is complex and may be multifactorial including any combination of: direct effects of conditioning chemotherapy and irradiation on bone cells, high-dose GCs, acquired GH deficiency or primary gonadal failure caused by the conditioning regimens, malabsorption caused by graft versus host disease and the underlying malignancy itself.

There is evidence for direct damage of the marrow stroma by the conditioning regimens used during BMT. Colony-forming units-fibroblasts (CFU-f) are the precursor compartment for the osteogenic lineage. In a mainly cross-sectional study of BMT survivors, Galotto et al. [49] reported that CFU-f frequencies were reduced by 60–90% following BMT, with no recovery up to 12 years after BMT. In a small group followed prospectively, all had zero CFU-f 20 days after BMT with no recovery up to 1 year, except in children younger than 5 years most of whom did show CFU-f recovery by 1 year after BMT. The marrow stromal microenvironment damage occurred regardless of the type of conditioning regimen and appeared to be irreversible in all except the youngest children.

Many reports in adults undergoing BMT have demonstrated acute decreases in bone formation markers and increases in bone resorption markers. Although bone formation markers return to normal after 3 months to 1 year, bone resorption markers may remain persistently increased for 1 year or more. This is associated with bone loss in the lumbar spine and hip, mainly occurring in the first 6 months, with a small proportion of patients developing vertebral compression fractures. A high proportion of survivors develop osteopenia or osteoporosis both in the lumbar spine and the hip. Survivors with the greatest depression in CFU-f have the lowest BMD z scores, indicating that inability to regenerate a normal number of osteoblastic precursors has a long-term adverse effect on bone mass [50].

Because BMT is performed relatively infrequently in the treatment of childhood cancer, fewer studies have been carried out in the paediatric age group. Table 3 shows details of four studies that have investigated BMD outcome following BMT in childhood. All showed significant reductions in lumbar spine or

Table 3. Cross-sectional studies of BMD outcome after BMT in childhood

Number of patients	Underlying diagnosis	Age at BMT years	Age at study years	Gender M/F	Length of follow-up from BMT years	Conditioning regimen	GVHD	aBMD by DEXA (z score)		LS trabecular vBMD by QCT (z score)	Reference
								total body	lumbar spine		
10	AML (9)[a] CML (1)	5 (3–18)	12 (4–22)	7/3	2 (1–10)	CP/TBI (1)[a] Bu/CP (8) Both (1)	6	–0.5 (–2.0 to +1.0)	–	–	51
25	ALL (21) AML (2) CML (1) NHL (1)	11 (6–18)	17 (11–26)	13/12	8 (4–13)	CP/TBI (25)	12	–0.5	–0.5	–	52
15	NS	NS	15 (9–18)	7/8	6 (1–12)	NS	NS	–0.9 (–3.6 to +1.8)	–0.9 (–2.8 to +2.8)	–	53
48	Cancer: ALL (10) AML (12) CML (9) MDS (9) Other (1) Non-cancer (5)	10 (1–20)	16 (4–27)	24/24	5 (1–10)	Cancer: CP/Cy/TBI Non-cancer: Bu/CP	28	–	–	–0.9 (–3.3 to +2.3)	54

GVHD = Graft versus host disease; LS = lumbar spine; ALL = acute lymphoblastic leukaemia; AML = acute myeloid leukaemia; CML = chronic myeloid leukaemia; MDS = myelodysplastic syndrome; CP = cyclophosphamide; Bu = busulphan; Cy = cytarabine; TBI = total body irradiation; NS = not stated.
Data are expressed as mean or median (range), where this information is provided.
[a] Number of patients.

total body BMD. This did not appear to be a consequence of reduced bone size as a result of poor growth because in one study BMAD was also low [53], and in another vertebral trabecular vBMD (by QCT) was low [54]. Indeed, in the latter study 21% survivors had vertebral trabecular BMD z scores below –2 and a further 26% had z scores between –2 and –1. Additionally, magnetic resonance imaging showed evidence of osteonecrosis in nearly half of all BMT survivors.

Petryk et al. [55] recently reported a prospective study on 49 children with various underlying disorders (23 cancer-related) undergoing BMT with a variety of conditioning regimens. They observed a significant reduction in lumbar spine aBMD and BMAD at 6 months and 1 year after BMT, although height z score showed no significant change. The proportion of patients with BMD z scores below –2 increased from 16% at baseline to 26% at 6 months and 19% at 1 year, whilst the proportion with BMD z scores between –2 and –1 increased from 18% at baseline to 33% at 6 months and 1 year. Patients with ALL or AML were at higher risk of bone loss in the first 6 months than other groups. The reduction in BMD at 6 months correlated with cumulative dose of GCs, with those who showed no recovery in BMD at 1 year having been exposed to higher doses. Bone ALP and osteocalcin (reflecting bone formation) decreased to a nadir at 3 months, then increased to above baseline whilst urinary N-telopeptide of type I collagen (bone resorption) showed a similar trend. Osteocalcin remained lower in those who showed no BMD recovery, probably reflecting the higher doses of GCs in this group.

To summarise, in children as in adults, there is evidence of long-term bone loss following BMT, especially at the lumbar spine, and mainly arising from inadequate osteoblast function. Children younger than 5 years may be less susceptible to these long-term adverse effects, but the evidence is sketchy. Osteonecrosis is also seen in a high proportion of survivors after BMT.

Long-Term Monitoring and Treatment to Optimise Bone Health in Childhood Cancer

Several studies have identified low physical activity and poor exercise capacity as risk factors for the development of low BMD in survivors of childhood cancer (see above). Improving ambulation and physical activity is clearly important in this group to optimise bone mass accrual during puberty, maximise peak bone mass and reduce bone loss.

As already discussed, cranial irradiation or total body irradiation may cause deficiencies of GH and other pituitary hormones. Although GH deficiency is the commonest abnormality, it may not always be easy to diagnose. In patients who have received 24 Gy or more, a combination of careful growth monitoring through childhood and puberty, regular measurements of IGF-1 (with interpretation against appropriate paediatric age-, gender- and assay-specific reference ranges) and provocative testing for GH may be required. The deleterious effects of GH deficiency on bone can be prevented by appropriate GH treatment, continuing into adulthood [32]. Long-term monitoring of TSH, free thyroxine, LH/FSH and oestradiol/testosterone is also required in survivors who have received 30 Gy or more of cranial irradiation, as deficits may occur several years after irradiation, with hormonal replacement as necessary. Similarly, all patients with Hodgkin's lymphoma who have received neck irradiation will require long-term monitoring of free thyroxine and TSH, with treatment of hypo- or less commonly hyperthyroidism as appropriate.

Long-term monitoring of LH/FSH and sex steroid is warranted in all patients who have received gonadal irradiation at doses exceeding the threshold for possible Leydig cell, germ cell or ovarian damage (see above and also separate chapters on male and female fertility after childhood cancer). Long-term monitoring is also required in both males and females who have received high doses of alkylating agents, including those administered as part of myeloablative BMT conditioning regimens, and in girls who have received cisplatin. If testosterone or oestradiol levels are low, accompanied by raised LH/FSH, pubertal induction and long-term androgen or oestrogen replacement is indicated, not only for sexual health but also to reduce the risk of developing osteoporosis. It is not yet established whether or not androgen treatment is beneficial in the case of compensated Leydig cell dysfunction when testosterone levels are normal but LH is increased.

Oestrogen replacement in adult female cancer survivors begs the question as to what form of hormone replacement is best. The choice generally lies between one of the oral contraceptive pills and low oestrogen hormone replacement therapy, as designed for much older post-menopausal women. Neither may be adequate for optimal bone health in young women with primary ovarian failure who face many years of oestrogen replacement.

Treatment of osteopenia directly caused by chemotherapy is a challenging and controversial topic. Bisphosphonates are a group of drugs that inhibit bone resorption through a variety of mechanisms and have been widely used in the treatment of post-menopausal osteoporosis. They have also been successfully used in the treatment of GC-induced osteoporosis in adults, with improvement in BMD at all skeletal sites and a substantial decrease in fracture risk. They may therefore be a candidate class of drugs for the treatment of osteopenia in children with cancer.

Pamidronate is a bisphosphonate that has been widely used for the treatment of severe symptomatic osteoporosis and osteogenesis imperfecta in children, with a good safety profile to date. In a small pilot study, 10 children with ALL were treated with intravenous infusions of pamidronate (1 mg/kg over 4 h on each of 3 successive days) during maintenance chemotherapy, repeated after 3 months [56]. The mean baseline lumbar spine aBMD z score was –1.9 (range –3.3 to –0.3) and appeared to improve over the 6-month study period. Unfortunately, 3 children were forced to withdraw owing to unacceptable side effects during infusions (severe hyperpyrexia and bilateral conjunctivitis), rendering pamidronate unsuitable for use in ALL patients. The same group of investigators have subsequently carried out another 6-month pilot study in children on maintenance chemotherapy for ALL or non-Hodgkin's lymphoma, this time using weekly oral alendronate as bisphosphonate therapy, together with calcium supplementation [57]. This time, tolerance was good and there were no significant side effects. Osteocalcin (bone formation marker) and CTx (bone resorption marker) both decreased sharply in the first week of treatment. Thereafter, mean osteocalcin remained above baseline whilst CTx remained below baseline, indicating a favourable balance of bone formation in relation to bone resorption. Mean whole body BMC z score was –1.9 (–4.7 to 0.0) at study entry and improved to –1.4 (–4.1 to +0.8) at 6 months. The mean lumbar spine aBMD z score increased from –1.3 (–2.7 to –0.3) to –0.8 (–1.9 to +0.7). Following these promising pilot study results, a full randomised control trial is required to confirm any benefit. It should be noted that, except in the context of a clinical trial, bisphosphonate treatment is not warranted in children based on aBMD measurements alone, unless there is also concurrent evidence of bone pathology (recurrent atraumatic fracture, bone pain). In children with ALL or other forms of cancer, this caveat is doubly important.

Conclusions

Children with cancer are exposed to multiple risk factors for the development of osteopenia, only some of which arise from endocrinopathy developing during or after treatment. Most clinical studies have concentrated on survivors of childhood ALL, partly because this is the commonest childhood cancer, partly because they form a relatively homogeneous group and partly because of the clinical impression that this group has the greatest fracture risk during and immediately after treatment. However, it must be borne in mind that ALL treatment protocols change through time and many outcome studies include children treated under different protocols. There is now good evidence that earlier protocols that included cranial irradiation with doses of 24 Gy or greater may result in deficiency of GH and lower BMD in the lumbar spine and femoral neck. How this relates to long-term fracture risk as this cohort of survivors ages remains to be ascertained.

Although there is little doubt that the intensive chemotherapy administered to children with ALL has adverse effects on bone, manifested by an increased fracture rate during treatment, the long-term consequences are still speculative. Children treated with chemotherapy alone are generally younger than those treated with earlier protocols that included cranial irradiation, with more limited follow-up. Some studies have reported normal BMD in this group but others have reported reduced BMD, especially at the lumbar spine. Again, there is no information as to how this may translate into long-term fracture risk. A pilot study has suggested that treatment with oral alendronate during the maintenance phase of ALL treatment may ameliorate the BMD deficit that arises during treatment. However, bisphosphonate treatment may carry increased risks of side effects in ALL patients and should not be contemplated outside the confines of a clinical trial until further evidence emerges.

The evidence relating to long-term bone health in children treated for solid tumours is patchy compared with ALL survivors. Patients with brain tumours often receive relatively high doses of cranial irradiation, with consequent pituitary hormone deficits, low BMD outcome and probable increased fracture risk. Survivors of childhood bone tumours also appear to have low BMD outcome, presumably relating to their chemotherapy and persisting well into adulthood. However, there is, as yet, little evidence regarding BMD outcome in survivors of other childhood cancers because the numbers are too few and treatments are too heterogeneous to reach firm conclusions.

Although there have been relatively few studies of survivors of childhood cancer who have received BMT, this group appears to be at greatly increased risk of osteopenia. The pathogenesis is likely to be multifactorial. Follow-up is as yet limited, so it is unknown whether any or all of these children will recover bone mass during adulthood.

References

1 Schoenau E, Saggese G, Peter F, Baroncelli GI, Shaw NJ, Crabtree NJ, Zadik Z, Neu CM, Noordam C, Radetti G, Hochberg Z: From bone biology to bone analysis. Horm Res 2004;61:257–269.

2 Sklar C: Endocrine complications of the successful treatment of neoplastic diseases in childhood. Growth Genet Horm 2001;17:37–42.

3 Bex M, Bouillon R: Growth hormone and bone health. Horm Res 2003;60(suppl 3):80–86.

4 Ahmed SR, Shalet SM, Beardwell CG: The effects of cranial irradiation on growth hormone secretion. Acta Paediatr Scand 1986;75:255–260.

5 Kirk JA, Raghupathy P, Stevens MM, Cowell CT, Mehnser MA, Bergin M, Tink A, Vines RH, Silink M: Growth failure and growth-hormone deficiency after treatment for acute lymphoblastic leukaemia. Lancet 1987;i:190–193.

6 Howell SJ, Radford JA, Adams JE, Shalet SM: The impact of mild Leydig cell dysfunction following cytotoxic chemotherapy on bone mineral density (BMD) and body composition. Clin Endocrinol (Oxf) 2000;52:609–616.

7 Siebler T, Shalet SM, Robson H: Effects of chemotherapy on bone metabolism and skeletal growth. Horm Res 2002;58(suppl 1):80–85.

8 Canalis E: Mechanisms of glucocorticoid action in bone: implications to glucocorticoid-induced osteoporosis. J Clin Endocrinol Metab 1996;81:3441–3447.

9 Weinstein RS, Jilka RL, Parfitt AM, Manolagas SC: Inhibition of osteoblastogenesis and promotion of apoptosis of osteoblasts and osteocytes by glucocorticoids. J Clin Invest 1998;102:274–282.

10 Schwartz AM, Leonidas JC: Methotrexate osteopathy. Skeletal Radiol 1984;11:13–16.

11 May KP, West SG, McDermott MT, Huffer WE: The effect of low-dose methotrexate on bone metabolism and histomorphometry in rats. Arthritis Rheum 1994;37:201–206.

12 Davies JH, Evans BAJ, Jenney MEM, Gregory JW: In vitro effects of chemotherapeutic agents on human osteoblast-like cells. Calcif Tissue Int 2002;70:408–415.

13 Davies JH, Evans BAJ, Jenney MEM, Gregory JW: Effects of chemotherapeutic agents on the function of primary human osteoblast-like cells derived from children. J Clin Endocrinol Metab 2003;88:6088–6097.

14 Crofton PM, Ahmed SF, Wade JC, Stephen R, Elmlinger MW, Ranke MB, Kelnar CJH, Wallace WHB: Effects of intensive chemotherapy on bone and collagen turnover and the growth hormone axis in children with acute lymphoblastic leukemia. J Clin Endocrinol Metab 1998;83:3121–3129.

15 Loebstein R, Atanackovic G, Bishai R, Wolpin J, Khattak S, Hashemi G, Gobrial M, Baruchel S, Ito S, Koren G: Risk factors for long-term outcome of ifosfamide-induced nephrotoxicity in children. J Clin Pharmacol 1999;39:454–461.

16 De Schepper J, Hachimi-Idrissi S, Louis O, Maurus R, Otten J: Bone metabolism and mineralization after cytotoxic chemotherapy including ifosfamide. Arch Dis Child 1994;71:346–348.

17 Robson H, Anderson E, Eden OB, Isaksson O, Shalet SM: Chemotherapeutic agents used in the treatment of childhood malignancies have direct effects on growth plate chondrocyte proliferation. J Endocrinol 1998;157:225–235.
18 Friedlaender GE, Tross RB, Doganis AC, Kirkwood JM, Baron R: Effects of chemotherapeutic agents on bone. I. Short-term methotrexate and doxorubicin (adriamycin) treatment in a rat model. J Bone Joint Surg Am 1984;66:602–607.
19 Robson H, Anderson E, Eden O, Isaksson O, Shalet S: Glucocorticoid pre-treatment reduces the cytotoxic effects of a variety of DNA-damaging agents on rat tibial growth-plate chondrocytes in vitro. Cancer Chemother Pharmacol 1998;42:171–176.
20 Halton JM, Atkinson SA, Fraher L, Webber CE, Cockshott WP, Tam C, Barr RD: Mineral homeostasis and bone mass at diagnosis in children with acute lymphoblastic leukemia. J Pediatr 1995;126:557–564.
21 Halton JM, Atkinson SA, Fraher L, Webber C, Gill GJ, Dawson S, Barr RD: Altered mineral metabolism and bone mass in children during treatment for acute lymphoblastic leukemia. J Bone Miner Res 1996;11:1774–1783.
22 Tragiannidis A, Athanassiadou F, Rousso I, Karamouzis M, Katzos G, Tsitouridis I, Sidi V, Koliouskas D: Evaluation of bone metabolism in children with acute lymphoblastic leukemia. A 2-year study from northern Greece. J Pediatr Hematol Oncol 2006;28:699.
23 Van der Sluis IM, van den Heuvel-Eibrink MM, Hählen K, Krenning EP, de Muinck Keizer-Schrama SMPF: Altered bone mineral density and body composition, and increased fracture risk in childhood acute lymphoblastic leukemia. J Pediatr 2002;141:204–210.
24 Sorva R, Kivivuori S-M, Turpeinen M, Marttinen E, Risteli J, Risteli L, Sorva A, Siimes MA: Very low rate of type I collagen synthesis and degradation in newly diagnosed children with acute lymphoblastic leukemia. Bone 1997;20:139–143.
25 Strauss AJ, Su JT, Kimball Dalton VM, Gelber RD, Sallan SE, Silverman LB: Bony morbidity in children treated for acute lymphoblastic leukemia. J Clin Oncol 2001;19:3066–3072.
26 Arikoski P, Komulainen J, Riikonen P, Jurvelin JS, Voutilainen R, Kröger H: Reduced bone density at completion of chemotherapy for a malignancy. Arch Dis Child 1999;80:143–148.
27 Crofton PM, Ahmed SF, Wade JC, Elmlinger MW, Ranke MB, Kelnar CJH, Wallace WHB: Bone turnover and growth during and after continuing chemotherapy in children with acute lymphoblastic leukemia. Pediatr Res 2000;48:490–496.
28 Brennan BM, Rahim A, Adams JA, Eden OB, Shalet SM: Reduced bone mineral density in young adults following cure of acute lymphoblastic leukaemia in childhood. Br J Cancer 1999;79:1859–1863.
29 Hoorweg-Nijman JJG, Kardos G, Roos JC, van Dijk HJ, Netelenbos C, Popp-Snijders C, de Ridder CM, Delemarre-van de Waal HA: Bone mineral density and markers of bone turnover in young adult survivors of childhood lymphoblastic leukaemia. Clin Endocrinol (Oxf) 1999;50:237–244.
30 Marinovic D, Dorgeret S, Lescoeur B, Alberti C, Noel M, Czernichow P, Sebag G, Vilmer E, Léger J: Improvement in bone mineral density and body composition in survivors of childhood acute lymphoblastic leukemia: a 1-year prospective study. Pediatrics 2005;116:e102–e108.
31 Warner JT, Evans WD, Webb DKH, Bell W, Gregory JW: Relative osteopenia after treatment for acute lymphoblastic leukemia. Pediatr Res 1999;45:544–551.
32 Nussey SS, Hyer SL, Brada M, Leiper AD: Bone mineralization after treatment of growth hormone deficiency in survivors of childhood malignancy. Acta Paediatr Suppl 1994;399:9–15.
33 Kaste SC, Jones-Wallace D, Rose SR, Boyett JM, Lustig RH, Rivera GK, Pui C-H, Hudson MM: Bone mineral decrements in survivors of childhood acute lymphoblastic leukemia: frequency of occurrence and risk factors for their development. Leukemia 2001;15:728–734.
34 Gilsanz V, Carlson ME, Roe TF, Ortega JA: Osteoporosis after cranial irradiation for acute lymphoblastic leukemia. J Pediatr 1990;117:238–244.
35 Arikoski P, Komulainen J, Voutilainen R, Riikonen P, Parviainen M, Tapanainen P, Knip M, Kröger H: Reduced bone mineral density in long-term survivors of childhood acute lymphoblastic leukemia. J Pediatr Hematol Oncol 1998;20:234–240.
36 Jarfelt M, Fors H, Lannering B, Bjarnason R: Bone mineral density and bone turnover in young adult survivors of childhood acute lymphoblastic leukaemia. Eur J Endocrinol 2006;154:303–309.
37 Mandel K, Atkinson S, Barr RD, Pencharz P: Skeletal morbidity in childhood acute lymphoblastic leukemia. J Clin Oncol 2004;22:1215–1221.

38 Nysom K, Holm K, Fleischer Michaelsen K, Hertz H, Müller J, Mølgaard C: Bone mass after treatment for acute lymphoblastic leukemia in childhood. J Clin Oncol 1998;16:3752–3760.
39 Van der Sluis IM, van den Heuvel-Eibrink MM, Hählen K, Krenning EP, de Muinck Keizer-Schrama SMPF: Bone mineral density, body composition, and height in long-term survivors of acute lymphoblastic leukemia in childhood. Med Pediatr Oncol 2000;35:415–420.
40 Tillmann V, Darlington ASE, Eiser C, Bishop NJ, Davies HA: Male sex and low physical activity are associated with reduced spine bone mineral density in survivors of childhood acute lymphoblastic leukemia. J Bone Miner Res 2002;17:1073–1080.
41 Brennan BMD, Mughal Z, Roberts SA, Ward K, Shalet SM, Eden OB, Will AM, Stevens RF, Adams JE: Bone mineral density in childhood survivors of acute lymphoblastic leukemia treated without cranial irradiation. J Clin Endocrinol Metab 2005; 90:689–694.
42 Kaste SC, Rai SN, Fleming K, McCammon EA, Tylavsky FA, Danish RK, Rose SR, Sitter CD, Pui C-H, Hudson MM: Changes in bone mineral density in survivors of childhood acute lymphoblastic leukemia. Pediatr Blood Cancer 2006;46: 77–87.
43 Van Beek RD, de Muinck Keizer-Schrama SMPF, Hakvoort-Cammel FG, Van der Sluis IM, Krenning EP, Pieters R, van den Heuvel-Eibrink MM: No difference between prednisolone and dexamethasone treatment in bone mineral density and growth in long term survivors of childhood acute lymphoblastic leukemia. Pediatr Blood Cancer 2006;46:88–93.
44 Arikoski P, Komulainen J, Riikonen P, Parviainen M, Jurvelin JS, Voutilainen R, Kröger H: Impaired development of bone mineral density during chemotherapy: a prospective analysis of 46 children newly diagnosed with cancer. J Bone Miner Res 1999;14:2002–2009.
45 Bath LE, Crofton PM, Evans AEM, Ranke MB, Elmlinger MW, Kelnar CJH, Wallace WHB: Bone turnover and growth during and after chemotherapy in children with solid tumours. Pediatr Res 2004;55:224–230.
46 Odame I, Duckworth J, Talsma D, Beaumont L, Furlong W, Webber C, Barr R: Osteopenia, physical activity and health-related quality of life in survivors of brain tumors treated in childhood. Pediatr Blood Cancer 2006;46:357–362.
47 Azcona C, Burghard E, Ruza E, Gimeno J, Sierrasesúmaga L: Reduced bone mineralization in adolescent survivors of malignant bone tumors: comparison of quantitative ultrasound and dual energy X-ray absorptiometry. J Pediatr Hematol Oncol 2003;25:297–302.
48 Holzer G, Krepler P, Koschat MA, Grampp S, Dominkus M, Kotz R: Bone mineral density in long-term survivors of highly malignant osteosarcoma. J Bone Joint Surg Br 2003;85:231–237.
49 Galotto M, Berisso G, Delfino L, Podesta M, Ottaggio L, Dallorso S, Dufour C, Ferrara GB, Abbondandolo A, Dini G, Bacigalupo A, Cancedda R, Quarto R: Stromal damage as consequence of high-dose chemo/radiotherapy in bone marrow transplant recipients. Exp Hematol 1999; 27:1460–1466.
50 Tauchmanovà L, Serio B, del Puente A, Risitano AM, Esposito A, de Rosa G, Lombardi G, Colao A, Rotoli B, Selleri C: Long-lasting bone damage detected by dual-energy X-ray absorptiometry, phalangeal osteosonogrammetry, and in vitro growth of marrow stromal cells after allogeneic stem cell transplantation. J Clin Endocrinol Metab 2002;87:5058–5065.
51 Bhatia S, Ramsay NKC, Weisdorf D, Griffiths H, Robison LL: Bone mineral density in patients undergoing bone marrow transplantation for myeloid malignancies. Bone Marrow Transplant 1998;22:87–90.
52 Nysom K, Holm K, Fleischer Michaelsen K, Hertz H, Jacobsen N, Müller J, Mølgaard C: Bone mass after allogeneic BMT for childhood leukaemia or lymphoma. Bone Marrow Transplant 2000;25: 191–196.
53 Daniels MW, Wilson DM, Paguntalan HG, Hoffman AR, Bachrach LK: Bone mineral density in pediatric transplant recipients. Transplantation 2003;76:673–678.
54 Kaste SC, Shidler TJ, Tong X, Srivastava DK, Rochester R, Hudson MM, Shearer PD, Hale GA: Bone mineral density and osteonecrosis in survivors of childhood allogeneic bone marrow transplantation. Bone Marrow Transplant 2004;33: 435–441.
55 Petryk A, Bergemann TL, Polga KM, Ulrich KJ, Raatz SK, Brown DM, Robison LL, Baker KS: Prospective study of changes in bone mineral density and turnover in children after hematopoietic cell transplantation. J Clin Endocrinol Metab 2006;91:899–905.

56 Barr RD, Guo CY, Wiernikowski J, Webber C, Wright M, Atkinson S: Osteopenia in children with acute lymphoblastic leukemia: a pilot study of amelioration with pamidronate. Med Pediatr Oncol 2002;39:44–46.

57 Wiernikowski JT, Barr RD, Webber C, Guo CY, Wright M, Atkinson SA: Alendronate for steroid-induced osteopenia in children with acute lymphoblastic leukaemia or non-Hodgkin's lymphoma: results of a pilot study. J Oncol Pharm Pract 2005;11:51–56.

Patricia M. Crofton, Honorary Senior Lecturer
Department of Paediatric Biochemistry, Royal Hospital for Sick Children, University of Edinburgh
Sciennes Road
Edinburgh EH9 1LF (UK)
Tel. +44 131 536 0403, Fax +44 131 536 0410, E-Mail patricia.crofton@luht.scot.nhs.uk

Wallace WHB, Kelnar CJH (eds): Endocrinopathy after Childhood Cancer Treatment.
Endocr Dev. Basel, Karger, 2009, vol 15, pp 101–134

Male Fertility and Strategies for Fertility Preservation following Childhood Cancer Treatment

R.T. Mitchell[a] · P.T.K. Saunders[a] · R.M. Sharpe[a] · C.J.H. Kelnar[b] · W.H.B. Wallace[b]

[a]MRC Human Reproductive Sciences Unit, Centre for Reproductive Biology, Queen's Medical Research Institute, and [b]Royal Hospital for Sick Children, University of Edinburgh, Edinburgh, UK

Abstract

Infertility in the male is a potential complication of childhood cancer treatment for long-term survivors. The risk is dependent primarily on the treatment used, but also on the underlying disease. Chemotherapy (especially alkylating agents) and radiotherapy, even in low doses, may damage the seminiferous epithelium and impair spermatogenesis in both children and adults. Leydig cell function and testosterone production are generally preserved after chemotherapy and low dose radiotherapy, whilst larger doses of radiotherapy may result in hypogonadism. Patients treated with potentially gonadotoxic treatments require regular multidisciplinary follow-up including assessment of puberty and gonadal function. Currently the only option available for fertility preservation in young males treated for cancer is semen cryopreservation. For pre-pubertal patients, techniques for fertility preservation remain theoretical and as yet unproven. These include hormonal manipulation of the gonadal environment before treatment, germ cell transplantation and testis xenografting, which have all shown promise in a variety of animal studies. Refinement of these techniques requires investigations in relevant animal models. In the present chapter we include data which suggest that the common marmoset *(Callithrix jacchus)* monkey, a New World primate, exhibits important parallels with human testicular development and may help us to understand why the pre-pubertal testis is vulnerable to effects of cytotoxic therapy on future fertility.

This chapter will describe the long-term effects of cancer treatment in childhood on male fertility. It will begin with an overview of male gonadal development with particular emphasis on the different stages in childhood, when variation in the hormonal and/or cellular environment may affect the response of the gonad to cytotoxic treatment and may also alter the effectiveness of strategies for preservation of fertility in these patients. It will then describe the direct and indirect effects of cytotoxic therapy on the testis and the possible mechanisms involved. It will end with a review of the potential strategies for preserving fertility in survivors of childhood cancer, including established techniques as well as those that are currently experimental. Throughout this chapter studies undertaken in animals will be discussed to provide insight into gonadal development, effects of cytotoxic therapy and fertility preservation, whilst relating these findings to the situation in the human. This will also serve to highlight differences between species that may result in different effects to those seen in humans.

Male Gonadal Axis and Gonad Development

The Male Reproductive Hormonal Axis

Secretion of gonadotropins from the pituitary gland is responsible for regulating hormonal control of the gonad in the male. Although this chapter will focus mainly on the gonad itself, knowledge of this central control of the gonad is particularly important for understanding the mechanisms behind the effects of cytotoxic therapy on fertility in addition to strategies for preserving fertility in survivors of childhood cancer.

The male hypothalamo-pituitary-gonadal axis (HPG) is active from fetal life and the level of hormones produced varies at different stages throughout life. The axis regulates the onset of puberty and the establishment of spermatogenesis, in addition to the production of gonadal androgens. Gonadotropin-releasing hormone (GnRH) is produced by the hypothalamus and stimulates the secretion of the gonadotropins in the form of luteinising hormone (LH) and follicle-stimulating hormone (FSH) from the anterior pituitary. LH acts on the testis to promote testosterone secretion from the Leydig cells and FSH acts on the Sertoli cells to initiate spermatogenesis. Two important negative feedback loops exist to regulate the secretion of gonadotropins. The testosterone negative feedback loop is established in fetal life and inhibits hypothalamic and pituitary production of GnRH and LH. Inhibin-B, produced by the Sertoli cell, exerts inhibitory effects on FSH secretion from the pituitary gland, however this negative feedback loop is only established at around puberty [1] (fig. 1).

Development of the Testis

Fetal Life and Early Infancy

During fetal life, the primordial germ cell population is thought to arise from a small group of cells in the epiblast. In humans the primordial germ cells migrate

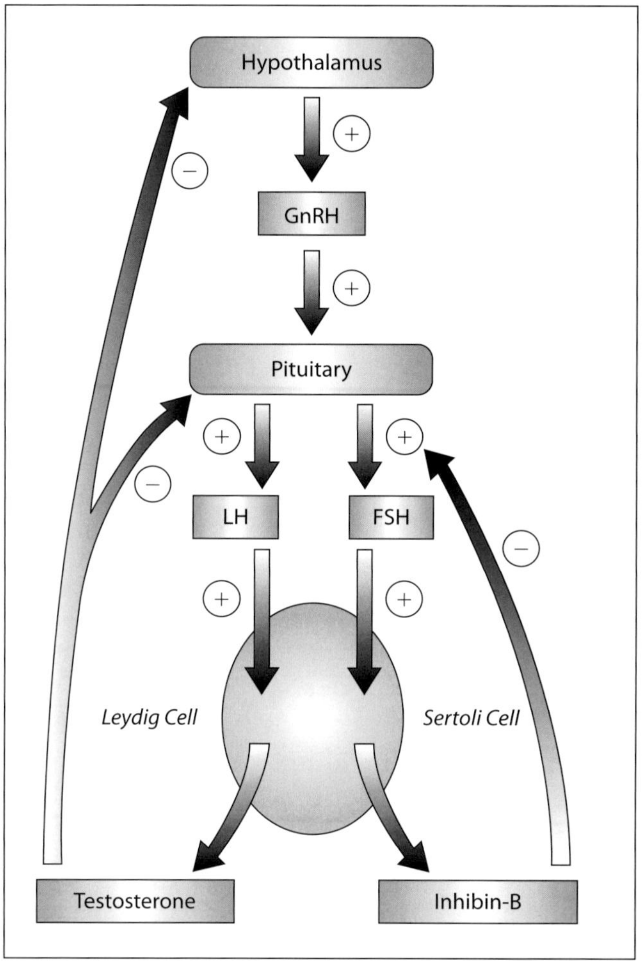

Fig. 1. The male hypothalamo-pituitary-gonadal axis. Stimulation (+) and inhibition (–) are indicated.

into the gonad during the 5th week of gestation and once they have become enclosed within seminiferous cords, they are termed gonocytes. These gonocytes begin to differentiate into spermatogonia and these in turn will ultimately give rise to spermatozoa at puberty. Also within the seminiferous epithelium are the Sertoli cells, which provide support to the developing germ cells. Leydig cells are located outside the seminiferous epithelium in the interstitial compartment and are responsible for producing androgens.

During infancy any remaining gonocytes will differentiate into spermatogonia. Differences exist between rodents and primates in terms of germ cell differentiation during this phase. In humans [2, 3] and primates such as the marmoset, gonocytes express protein markers associated with pluripotent or

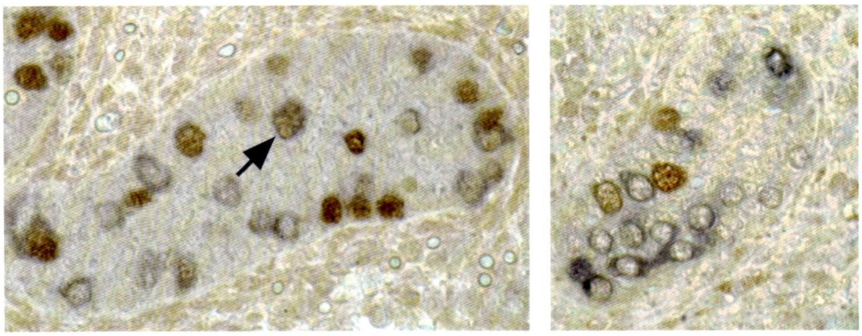

Fig. 2. Expression of OCT4 (brown) and VASA (blue) in marmoset testes from fetal (17/20 weeks gestation) and neonatal (1 day postnatal) animals. Note the progression within the cords, as the proportion of germ cells expressing OCT4 decreases and the proportion of germ cells expressing VASA increases. Cells express both markers (arrow) as they differentiate from OCT4 to VASA-positive germ cells.

undifferentiated germ cells such as OCT4 [2, 3] and AP-2γ [4]. These cells differentiate to become spermatogonia, during which the expression of these markers is gradually reduced and germ cell-specific markers such as VASA [2, 5] and MAGE-A4 [3, 4] are expressed (fig. 2). Rodents demonstrate a homogeneous population of cells expressing markers such as OCT4 and VASA simultaneously and become negative for OCT4 in a synchronous manner without the gradual transition seen in the human and primate. A potential consequence of the mixed population of gonocytes in the primate may be differences in the effects of cytotoxic therapy, when compared to rodents. This may be particularly relevant if cancer treatment begins during infancy, when differentiation of gonocytes is still occurring.

Following birth in humans and non-human primates there is an initial rise in gonadotropins and testosterone that continues during early infancy, the so-called 'mini puberty'. In humans the rise begins at 2 weeks of life and peaks between 1 and 3 months of age, falling to low levels at 6–8 months. This pattern of secretion has also been demonstrated in many other primates, including the rhesus monkey and the marmoset [6] (fig. 3).

Childhood

In humans and non-human primates after the rise in gonadotropins and testosterone during early infancy, there follows a period of relative 'quiescence' during which levels of these hormones are relatively low [6]. This period will be referred to as the 'childhood period', which lasts from the end of infancy until the onset of puberty (fig. 3). In rodents GnRH synthesis and release is not interrupted by a post-infantile quiescent period prior to the onset of puberty, which highlights

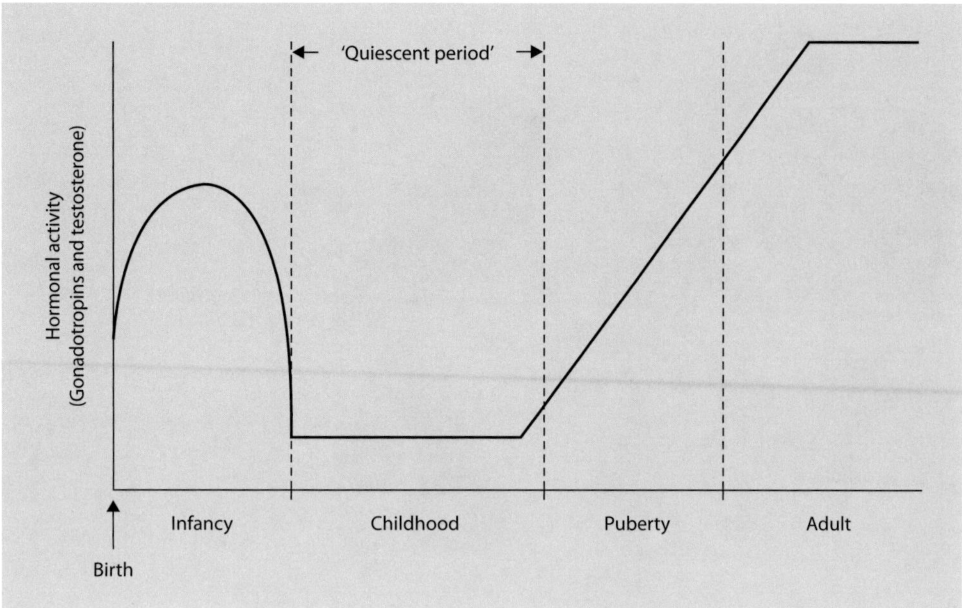

Fig. 3. The profile of gonadotropin and testosterone secretion in primates throughout life [6].

another fundamental difference between rodents and primates that may affect the response to cancer treatment.

Based on these low levels of gonadotropins and testosterone in primates, it had been assumed that the 'childhood' testis is a relatively quiescent organ and as a result, little germ cell proliferation occurred. As proliferating cells are considered to be the main targets of cancer therapy, in theory this should render the gonad less susceptible to the damaging effects of cytotoxic therapy. However the fact that gonadal damage occurs following cancer treatment in childhood raises doubt about whether the testis is truly quiescent during childhood. Studies have demonstrated in the human that there is pulsatile secretion of LH during sleep in mid-childhood which increases in amplitude prior to puberty [7], and that this is paralleled by incomplete spermatogenic bursts [8]. Demonstration of this activity raised the possibility that germ cell proliferation may occur in the testis during childhood and that this may render the gonad susceptible to damage by cancer treatment. To investigate this hypothesis, germ cell proliferation has been studied in the marmoset monkey during the 'childhood' period [9]. Immunohistochemical labelling using proliferating cell nuclear antigen showed that a proportion of germ cells are proliferating during this period [9]. A proliferation index obtained using Ki67 as the marker of mitotic activity has confirmed the presence of proliferating germ cells from birth through to adulthood in this primate species, with a lower proliferation index during the childhood period (fig. 4). This is also the

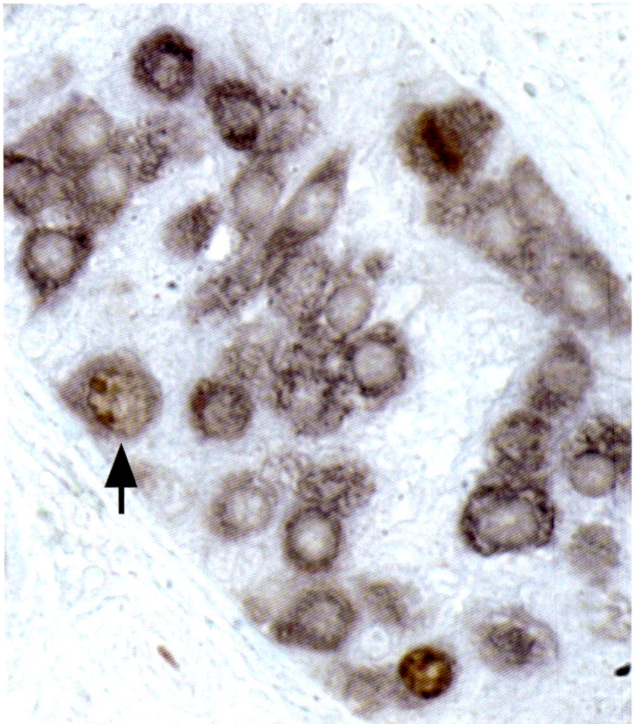

Fig. 4. Expression of VASA (blue) and Ki67 (brown) in a testis from a 35-week-old ('childhood') marmoset demonstrates the presence of proliferating germ cells (arrow) during the 'quiescent' phase of gonadotropin and testosterone secretion.

case for the human with proliferation of germ cells occurring during the childhood period. Ki67 expression has been demonstrated in 10.9% of human germ cells between the age of 1 and 6 years [10]. In the rat there is a block in G_0 of the cell cycle from late gestation until postnatal day 3–6, when proliferation resumes [11], indicating another potentially important difference between the primate and the rodent, which may have relevance for susceptibility to gonadal damage following cancer treatment.

Suppression of germ cell proliferation could in theory protect the gonad from the damaging effects of cytotoxic treatment. If germ cell proliferation is gonadotropin- or sex steroid-dependent, then the use of a GnRH antagonist might represent one strategy to achieve this. However treatment with a GnRH antagonist did not affect germ cell proliferation in the marmoset during the 'childhood' phase [9]. Indeed even treatment of marmosets with a GnRH antagonist during the neonatal period, when the levels of gonadotropins and testosterone are high, failed to have a major impact on germ cell proliferation, which remained at 70% of the control level (unpublished). This lack of complete suppression of proliferation by

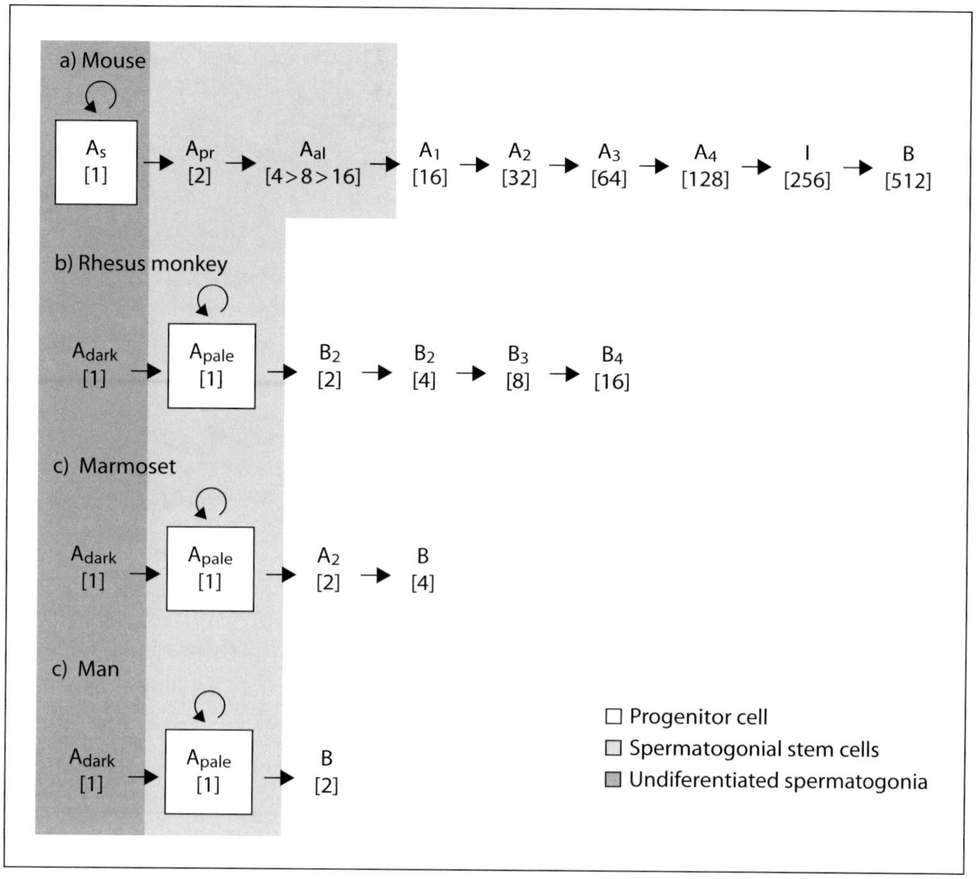

Fig. 5. Differences in spermatogonial sub-types and potential number of cells generated (brackets) between species. Adapted from Jahnukainen et al. [12].

a GnRH antagonist suggests that there are factors other than gonadotropins and testosterone involved in controlling germ cell proliferation and this will be important when, later in the chapter, we consider hormonal manipulation of the gonad to preserve fertility.

The germ cell population during the childhood phase consists of spermatogonia. There are different subtypes of spermatogonia within species and a variation between species (fig. 5). An important feature in primates is that the $A_{(dark)}$ spermatogonia are thought to be the spermatogonial stem cell and to act as the regenerative reserve, while $A_{(pale)}$ spermatogonia are the progenitor cells acting as the functional reserve [12]. However, in the mouse $A_{(single)}$ spermatogonia are considered to be the stem cell and it is suggested that the $A_{(single)}$ spermatogonia act as both the stem cell and the progenitor cell [12]. The cells most susceptible to cytotoxic therapy are those that are rapidly dividing. As the spermatogonial stem cells have a lower rate of proliferation than differentiated spermatogonia, it follows that these cells may be relatively protected compared to other germ cell types. Indeed it has been demonstrated that in the mouse undifferentiated spermatogonia are less sensitive to radiation than are differentiating spermatogonia [13].

Differences also exist in the theoretical numbers of germ cells that can result from each step of differentiation. More mitotic divisions of spermatogonia occur in the mouse compared to primates with the potential for the production of many more differentiated spermatogonia. In reality the theoretical numbers are not achieved because of apoptosis of a large proportion of the spermatogonial population [14].

The differences in spermatogonial subtype, function and number within individuals at different stages and between species may result in variable responses to cytotoxic therapy and impact on attempts to prevent them.

Puberty and Adulthood

The potential for future fertility following cancer treatment is difficult to assess in childhood because it depends on progression through puberty and establishment of spermatogenesis. Spermatogenesis is the process via which male spermatogonia proliferate and then differentiate into mature spermatozoa. This process is initiated by FSH during puberty and both FSH and testosterone appear to be required for normal spermatogenesis [14]. Testosterone acts via the androgen receptor on the Sertoli cell, exerting indirect effects on the germ cells.

Spermatogenesis can be divided into three phases that are common to all mammals [14]. During the proliferative or spermatogonial phase the spermatogonia undergo frequent mitotic divisions and form primary spermatocytes. This is followed by the meiotic phase, during which the tetraploid primary spermatocytes become diploid secondary spermatocytes. These secondary spermatocytes undergo the second meiotic division to become haploid spermatids. Spermiogenesis is the third phase when the spermatids differentiate into mature spermatozoa (fig. 6).

The seminiferous tubule is organised with the spermatogonia adjacent to the basement membrane. As the germ cells differentiate they are directed towards the lumen (fig. 7). Supporting the germ cells are the Sertoli cells which form the 'blood testis barrier' consisting of tight (occluding) junctions between adjacent Sertoli cells. Each Sertoli cell provides support for numerous germ cells at different stages of development and the function of the Sertoli cells at a given stage is determined by its germ cell complement [14]. Spermatogenesis can be classified according to the patterns of germ cell association from basement membrane to the tubule lumen. These are known as the stages of the spermatogenic cycle. In

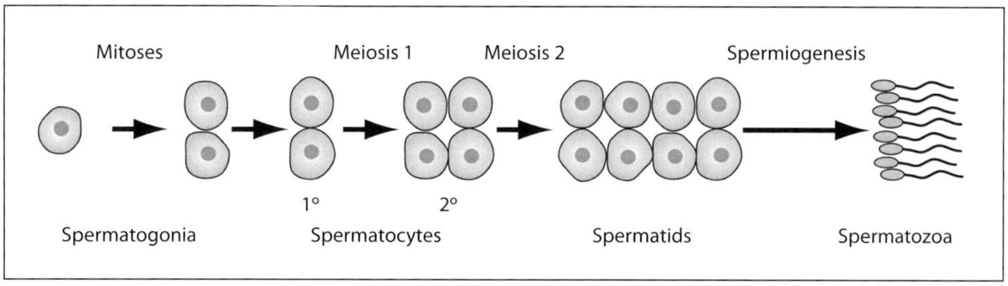

Fig. 6. Overview of mammalian spermatogenesis.

the human there are six such stages and each tubule cross-section will contain between one and five stages [15]. The marmoset also demonstrates multiple stages within a tubular cross-section [16]. In contrast a single stage of spermatogenesis is usually present in any cross-section of a rodent testis as well as in some non-human primates, such as the rhesus macaque [16].

It is likely that the differences in organisation of spermatogenesis, variation in germ cell complement and interaction with the supporting Sertoli cells, in addition to the hormonal environment may influence not only the effects of cytotoxic treatment in childhood, but also the potential for preservation of fertility for these patients. These differences between species are important and are considered below.

Effects of Cancer Treatment on Male Reproductive Function

Cytotoxic therapy may result in a number of effects on the male reproductive system in long-term survivors. These include direct effects on the seminiferous epithelium and indirect effects via damage to the hypothalamus or pituitary (fig. 8). In addition to these effects there may be others, such as obstruction of sperm transport, erectile dysfunction, consequences of disease, or the psychological effects of childhood cancer treatment and its effect on future relationships. Currently, despite advances in assisted reproduction, unless the patient can produce mature germ cells then reproductive potential cannot be preserved. Therefore the remainder of this chapter will focus mainly on the seminiferous epithelium and the production of mature germ cells.

The scale of the problem regarding future fertility in children treated for cancer is illustrated by a study which followed up children, between 2 and 16 years of age and diagnosed with various cancers, and found azoospermia in 30% of patients, whilst a further 18% were rendered oligozoospermic a median of 11.6 years after treatment [17].

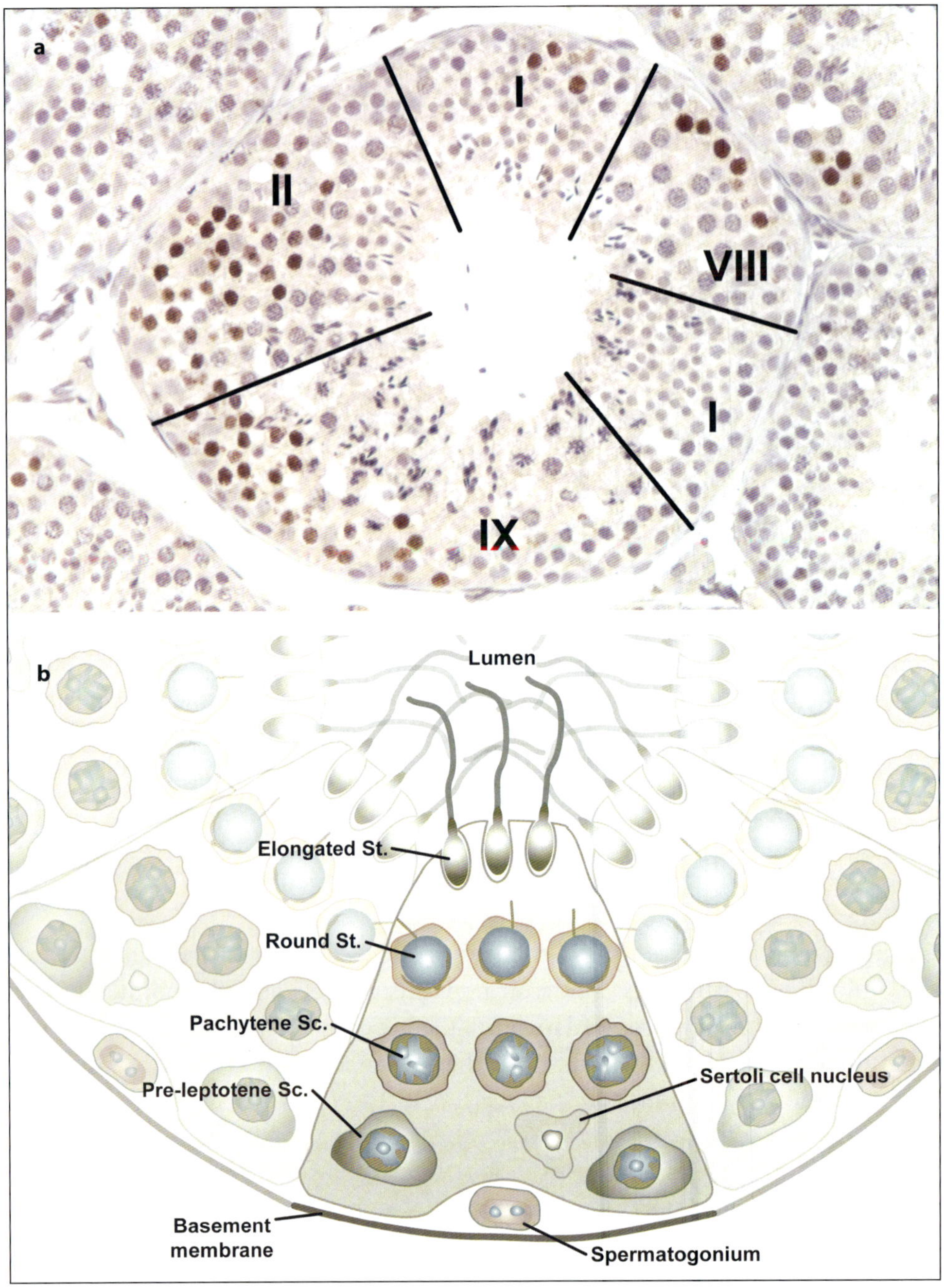

Fig. 7. Cross-section through a seminiferous tubule in a marmoset testis (**a**) and a schematic representation of a transverse view of a human seminiferous tubule (**b**). I, II, VIII and IX are stages of the seminiferous cycle. Sc. = Spermatocyte; St. = spermatid.

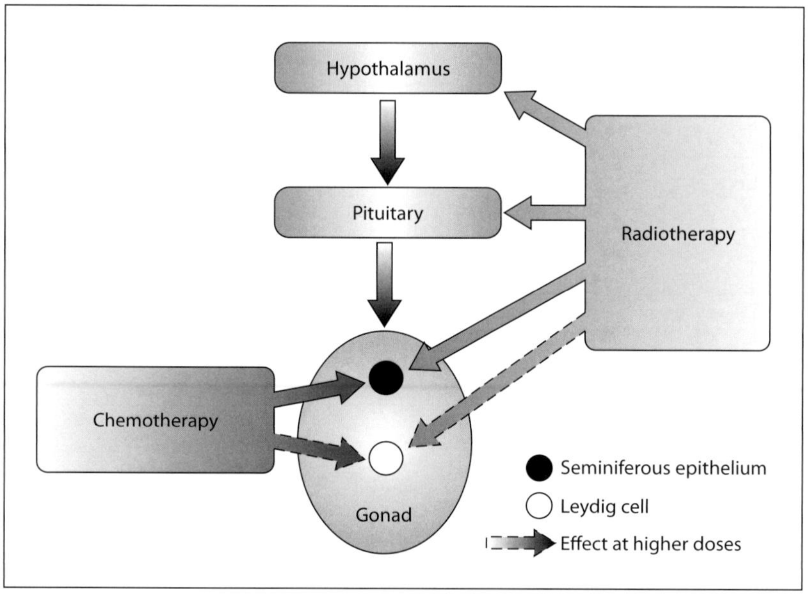

Fig. 8. Potential targets for impairment of fertility following chemotherapy and/or radiotherapy.

Effects of Cancer Treatment on the Gonad

Cytotoxic therapy may result in damage to the gonad, particularly with radiation to the gonad, total body irradiation or high dose chemotherapy (especially alkylating agents) [18] (table 1).

Radiotherapy

The effect of radiotherapy depends on the dose, treatment field and fractionation schedule [19]. Low doses of radiation may result in damage to the seminiferous epithelium, affecting spermatogonia and leading to oligozoospermia [20], whilst higher doses (>20 Gy) may also affect the Leydig cells, resulting in reduced serum testosterone and raised serum gonadotrophins. A study in children and young adults treated for Hodgkin's lymphoma, demonstrated a reduced testicular volume in 66% of patients and increased FSH in 87% of patients, indicative of damage to the seminiferous epithelium [21]. In contrast only 17% of patients had raised LH and 50% had reduced testosterone, supporting the idea that the Leydig cell is less sensitive to cytotoxic damage than the seminiferous epithelium.

Recovery of spermatogenesis is observed after low dose single fraction radiotherapy of 2–4 Gy [22], whilst doses of 6 Gy have been associated with azoospermia lasting at least 2 years [23]. These controversial studies involved irradiating the testes of participants who were described as healthy volunteers from the

Table 1. Gonadotoxic therapies used in the treatment of childhood cancers

Radiotherapy
Radiotherapy to field including testes
Total body irradiation
Chemotherapy
Alkylating agents
Cyclophasphamide
Ifosfamide
Nitrosureas, e.g. carmustine and lomustine
Chlorambucil
Melphalan
Busulphan
Cisplatin
Cytarabine
Dacarbazine
Procarbazine

prison population. Direct radiotherapy to the testis may involve doses as high as 20–24 Gy which results in eradication of germ cells [24] and causes permanent azoospermia [23]. Spermatogonia have been reported to be more radiosensitive than spermatocytes and spermatids with doses as low as 0.1 Gy causing damage to spermatogonia, while higher doses may affect spermatocytes and spermatids. This results in a faster fall in sperm concentration in those receiving a higher dose of radiation due to the loss of more mature germ cell types [25].

In clinical practice, fractionated radiotherapy is often used and this may also result in damage to the seminiferous epithelium [26]. Gonadal recovery in men treated with fractionated total body irradiation has been reported to occur in less than 20% of patients [27].

Chemotherapy

All chemotherapeutic drugs may have some effect on fertility, although some of these agents are known to be more gonadotoxic than others (table 1). The most gonadotoxic cytostatic agents are procarbazine and the alkylating agents, particularly cyclophosphamide. Treatment of the most common form of childhood cancer, acute lymphoblastic leukaemia, has been shown to result in damage to the seminiferous epithelium [28] and may be associated with the use of cyclophosphamide or cis-platinum [29]. The effects depend on the precise combination of drugs and the doses administered, in addition to the frequency/duration of administration. The combination of cyclophosphamide and busulphan as conditioning treatment for bone marrow transplant has been associated with a <20% chance of spermatogonial recovery [27]. In addition to adults, pre-pubertal patients are also susceptible to chemotherapy-induced damage to the seminiferous epithelium, particularly with treatment for Hodgkin's lymphoma. A study of the cumulative dose of cyclophosphamide required to result in permanent sterility in young male patients treated with combination therapy for Ewing and soft tissue sarcomas, suggested a dose of 7.5 g/m^2 [30] and a review by the National Cancer Institute led to the consensus that males who receive <4 g/m^2 of cyclophosphamide without any other alkylating agents and without either testicular or cranial irradiation are likely to retain their fertility. In patients receiving cumulative doses of cisplatin >400 mg/m^2, irreversible impairment of spermatogenic function should be expected [31].

Risk Categories for Specific Regimens

The risk of gonadal damage from individual drugs may not be as relevant to each patient as the overall treatment regimen used. On that basis the risk of sub-fertility can be divided into three categories (table 2). Low risk treatment (<20%) includes patients being treated for acute lymphoblastic leukaemia, the most common childhood malignancy. High risk treatment (>80%) includes total body irradiation or treatment of Hodgkin's lymphoma with alkylating agents [18].

The Mechanism of Gonadal Damage following Childhood Cancer Treatment

Understanding the mechanism of damage to the gonads during childhood cancer treatment is crucial for devising strategies to preserve reproductive function in these patients. Effects on germ, Sertoli or Leydig cells may result in reduced gonadal function. Direct effects on germ cells will interfere with spermatogenesis, whilst effects on the supporting Sertoli cells will indirectly affect germ cells and hence spermatogenesis. Recovery of spermatogenesis with return of sperm production may occur several years after treatment [30]. Effects on Leydig cells may result in failure to produce testosterone, which is required for initiation and maintenance of spermatogenesis and the development of secondary sexual characteristics. Because the effects of cytotoxic treatment within the human testis cannot be studied easily animal models are required.

Rodent studies have shown that the severity and duration of long-term fertility impairment following cytotoxic treatment correlates to the number of type A spermatogonia that are destroyed [31] and that the initiation and recovery from impaired spermatogenesis can therefore be predicted by the kinetics of the spermatogenic cycle [32]. In rodents it has been demonstrated that the resting spermatogonial stem cells are resistant to the effects of the cytotoxic agent busulphan because of cell cycle arrest. In irradiated rats the surviving spermatogonia are able

Table 2. Best assessment of risk of sub-fertility after current treatment for common cancers in childhood and adolescence [18]

Low risk (<20%)
Acute lymphoblastic leukaemia
Wilms' tumour
Soft-tissue sarcoma: stage 1
Germ cell tumours (with gonadal preservation and no radiotherapy)
Retinoblastoma
Brain tumour: surgery only, cranial irradiation <24 Gy
Medium risk
Acute myeloblastic leukaemia (difficult to quantify)
Hepatoblastoma
Osteosarcoma
Ewing's sarcoma: non-metastatic
Soft-tissue sarcoma: stage II or III
Neuroblastoma
Non-Hodgkin's lymphoma
Hodgkin's lymphoma: alternating treatment
Brain tumour: craniospinal radiotherapy, cranial irradiation >24 Gy
High risk (>80%)
Total body irradiation
Localised radiotherapy: pelvic or testicular
Chemotherapy conditioning for bone-marrow transplantation
Hodgkin's lymphoma: treatment with alkylating drugs
Soft tissue sarcoma: stage IV (metastatic)
Ewing's sarcoma: metastatic

to proliferate after cytotoxic exposure but undergo apoptosis when they are ready to differentiate [33]. This block of differentiation occurs 6 weeks after irradiation. Irradiation also leads to an increase in intra-testicular testosterone levels and subsequently to an increase in interstitial fluid volume and it has been postulated that this testicular oedema may be involved in the block of spermatogonial differentiation [34]. In addition to the increase in testicular testosterone levels, it has also been shown that procarbazine-treated or irradiated rats have elevated levels of FSH. This led to the hypothesis that elevated hormone levels may be inhibiting recovery of spermatogenesis [35]. This forms the basis for experiments that have involved manipulating the hormonal environment within the testis, which will be discussed in the next section.

In humans and non-human primates, a lack of germ stem cells is the likely cause for permanent absence of spermatogenic recovery, as opposed to the block of differentiation that occurs in rats [36]. Primate studies demonstrate that chemotherapy and radiation causes an initial depletion of differentiating spermatogonia in the adult gonad [37]. There is an initial decrease in the differentiating $A_{(pale)}$ spermatogonia, followed by an increase in $A_{(pale)}$ and decrease in $A_{(dark)}$ spermatogonia as the latter are activated into $A_{(pale)}$ cells. After this there is a decrease in numbers of both types of spermatogonia which is thought to be due to damage by irradiation of the $A_{(dark)}$ cells, such that the resulting $A_{(pale)}$ cells degenerate when attempting to divide. Subsequent recovery may occur and may be due to the activation of the surviving spermatogonial stem cells which are less proliferative and therefore withstand the treatment more effectively [12]. The lag phase would represent the time taken for the surviving stem cells to undergo a cycle of spermatogenesis. Lower doses of irradiation (0.5 Gy) in the rhesus monkey have been shown to result in faster recovery in terms of spermatogonial numbers when compared to doses of 1 or 2 Gy [38].

One long-term follow-up study has looked at the effects of irradiation with 4–8.5 Gy on the testes of pre-pubertal rhesus monkeys 3–8 years after treatment [39]. This resulted in complete loss of germ cells in some of the tubules in every animal studied. At the higher doses there were some animals with no repopulation of the tubules. There was also a significant reduction in testis weight, an increase in serum FSH and a reduction in inhibin B levels, consistent with Sertoli cell damage. At this age Sertoli cell numbers appear to be fixed and loss of Sertoli cells cannot be compensated by changes in proliferation or apoptosis [39]. Even at the highest dose (8.5 Gy) there was no effect on Leydig cell function.

Men rendered azoospermic by cancer therapy have significantly higher FSH and lower inhibin B than those that are non-azoospermic [17]. There may also be a decrease in testis weight or sperm count and biopsy of the testis post-treatment may demonstrate impaired spermatogenesis [28]. Effects on the production of testosterone from Leydig cells are only apparent at much higher doses. This means that patients treated pre-pubertally may develop secondary sexual characteristics normally despite the fact that there may be effects on spermatogenesis. The doses required to cause Leydig cell failure will invariably have resulted in damage to the seminiferous epithelium.

Other Effects on Fertility, Including Indirect Effects

Cranial irradiation may result in damage to the hypothalamo-pituitary axis with resulting downstream effects on gonadal function and fertility. Gonadotropin deficiency is the second most common pituitary hormone abnormality after growth hormone, following cranial irradiation. In the short term, doses of 30–50 Gy are known to cause precocious puberty in some patients, more frequently in young girls than boys, whilst doses of at least 30 Gy may infrequently result in true gonadotropin deficiency in the longer term [40]. In a study of 45 children treated with hypothalamic and pituitary radiation, severe gonadotropin deficiency was observed in 11% of cases, resulting in lack of or slow progression of puberty and decreased LH and FSH responsiveness to GnRH [41]. Studies in post-pubertal patients have demonstrated that in some the serum levels of testosterone are reduced and LH and FSH levels may be low. However demonstration of a pituitary response to GnRH [42] and growth hormone-releasing hormone [43], following cranial irradiation, suggests initial hypothalamic hypogonadism with pituitary insufficiency occurring later. There are also potential direct effects of the tumour. In the case of cranial malignancy there may also be damage to the axis as a result of invasion of the pituitary or hypothalamus with tumour or a pressure effect of the tumour on these structures. Surgery for these malignancies may also result in damage, in particular in the case of malignancies in close proximity to the hypothalamus or pituitary, such as craniopharyngioma. Management of potential gonadotropin insufficiency requires assessment of pubertal progression and hypothalamo-pituitary function, with replacement of gonadotropins or testosterone if necessary.

There are several other factors that may affect the reproductive potential in patients treated in childhood for cancer. It has been shown that impaired semen quality may exist in up to 70% of male patients prior to treatment for Hodgkin's lymphoma [44] and that abnormal spermatogenesis may exist in the majority of young patients with germ cell tumours prior to treatment [45]. Other physical effects of the disease itself such as pain, pyrexia or anorexia may also affect semen quality [18].

Follow-Up of Patients at Risk of Impaired Gonadal Function following Childhood Cancer Treatment

Predicting the likelihood of gonadal dysfunction in the individual patient may be difficult. Measurements of gonadotropins and testosterone in pre-pubertal patients will not be informative. The assessment of growth and puberty is very important and information on the presence of secondary sexual characteristics will provide information on testosterone production. Should Leydig cell function be significantly affected then delayed puberty may result. Testicular volumes may also indicate effects on the seminiferous epithelium, which may result in failure of normal spermatogenesis as evidenced by raised FSH and low inhibin B levels in patients with a testicular volume of <10 ml after the onset of puberty. Follow-up of patients requires a multi-disciplinary approach.

Many guidelines exist for long-term follow-up of children treated for cancer, with different strategies adopted between and also within individual countries.

Table 3. Options for preserving fertility in young males treated for cancer

Established
Shielding testes from irradiation
Modification of treatment regime
Cryopreservation of semen
Experimental
Hormonal manipulation of the gonadal environment
Cryopreservation
Germ cells
Testicular tissue
Xenografting
Germ cells
Testicular tissue

The assessment of male pubertal development and fertility may include: (1) assessment of testicular volume using the Prader orchidometer; (2) Tanner staging of secondary sexual development; (3) measurement of serum FSH, LH, testosterone and inhibin B (if available); (4) semen analysis; (5) men who have evidence of impaired fertility should be referred for specialist assessment as they could benefit from assisted reproductive techniques (ARTs); (6) fertility counselling should be provided to survivors of childhood cancer, and (7) cryopreservation of semen should be offered to young male patients whose cancer therapy will include potentially gonadotoxic treatments.

Preservation of Reproductive Potential following Childhood Cancer Treatment

Strategies to preserve fertility in young people treated for cancer are summarised in table 3. The first line of protection is to reduce exposure of the gonad to these agents. Secondly the treatment itself may be modified to reduce potential gonadal toxicity. For pubertal patients who are likely to suffer effects on fertility, semen cryopreservation can be offered; however, in patients unable to produce mature gametes, alternative strategies must be devised. Current research focuses on the possibility of hormonal protection of the gonad, long-term storage of testicular material or xenotransplantation into a host species. Transplanted material may subsequently be re-introduced into the patient or gametes may be extracted for ARTs such as in vitro fertilisation. The final section of this chapter will discuss these options in more detail.

Protective Measures

Methods to protect the gonad from direct damage such as limitation of radiation exposure by shielding of the testes should be practiced where possible [20].

Modification of Treatment Regimens for Childhood Cancer

Reduction in the dose and frequency of cytotoxic treatment, or substitution with a less gonadotoxic agent may all reduce the chances of gonadal damage. The changing treatment of Hodgkin's lymphoma is an example of how modification of treatment can attenuate the risk of gonadal dysfunction.

In a study of 355 adult patients with Hodgkin's lymphoma [46] treated with a regimen of either radiotherapy or non-alkylating agent chemotherapy, impaired spermatogenesis was demonstrated in 3 and 8% of patients, respectively (using elevated FSH as a proxy for impaired spermatogenesis). In contrast, 60% of patients treated with alkylating agent chemotherapy had impaired spermatogenesis. Recovery of spermatogenesis occurred in 82% of patients treated with non-alkylating agent chemotherapy after a median time of 19 months, whilst in patients receiving alkylating agents, recovery was demonstrated in 30% fewer patients.

In another study comparing two regimens of treatment, men treated with a regimen containing alkylating agents known as MOPP (chlormethine, procarbazine, vincristine and prednisolone), were shown to have persistent azoospermia in 86% of cases, whereas all patients treated with ABVD (doxorubicin, vinblastine, bleomycin and dacarbazine) demonstrated recovery of spermatogenesis [47]. Current treatment of children with Hodgkin's lymphoma in the UK aims to preserve fertility by avoiding exposure of the patient to procarbazine for low stage disease. A new comparative study in children and young people (<18 years) with Hodgkin's lymphoma is about to open, which will randomise patients with intermediate and high stage disease to a regimen that replaces procarbazine with dacarbazine. The aim of this study is to examine the safety of removing of procarbazine from the chemotherapy regimen and whether this affects the development of impaired fertility in these patients.

Cryopreservation of Semen

At present the only established method for preserving reproductive potential in patients who have already achieved full spermatogenesis is with cryopreservation of semen. This can be achieved by masturbation, penile vibratory stimulation or electrostimulation under anaesthetic, however the motility and sperm count may be reduced when the latter method is used [48]. Other techniques include epididymal aspiration and testicular biopsy; however the risk of compromising testicular function questions the suitability of the latter technique. The British Fertility Society recommendations are that all post-pubertal patients requiring treatment for cancer should be offered sperm banking. Semen cryopreservation is governed by the Human Fertilisation and Embryology Act, which states that written, informed consent by the individual must be obtained prior to semen cryopreservation and that they must understand the implications of what is proposed [18].

Despite recommendations, the option of sperm banking is not always offered. Reasons for failing to offer this treatment included cost, lack of facilities and a poor prognosis from the underlying condition [49]. When patients were offered sperm banking only 50% of them banked sperm, with lack of information cited as the most common reason for failing to bank [50]. Access to sperm banking is widespread in the UK and a study of patients aged between 13 and 21 showed that sperm banking was discussed with 91% of patients, resulting in sperm banking in 71% of cases [51]. Even when sperm banking is undertaken the number of resultant births may be low. In a study of patients about to receive treatment for Hodgkin's lymphoma, 115 men banked semen, 33 had utilised their semen after a median of 10 years and 11 live births occurred [52].

Hormonal Manipulation

One strategy to preserve fertility in patients treated for cancer involves manipulation of the gonadal environment to render the testis less susceptible to cytotoxic therapy. An initial hypothesis was that suppression of the HPG axis prior to cytotoxic therapy using agents such as sex steroids, GnRH antagonists or GnRH agonists would protect the gonad from cytotoxic damage. GnRH agonists cause initial stimulation of gonadotropin secretion, whilst repeated administration of GnRH agonist leads to HPG suppression by binding to the GnRH receptor and inhibiting production of gonadotropin and testosterone. There have been several promising studies in rodents that have demonstrated protection of spermatogenesis when hormonal suppression is commenced before treatment. It has also been shown that recovery of spermatogenesis can be enhanced when hormonal suppression is induced during and after treatment. This approach has so far failed to translate successfully into primates, including humans, and the relevant studies are summarised below.

Hormonal Manipulation of the Adult Rodent Testis

Pre-Cytotoxic Therapy. Treatment of adult rats for 6 weeks with testosterone and oestradiol, prior to irradiation, results in a higher germ cell repopulation index and sperm head count, compared to rats receiving irradiation alone [53]. Similar results were obtained with rats receiving procarbazine treatment [54]. Treatment of rats with GnRH agonist prior to procarbazine treatment has also resulted in a higher stem cell index and subsequent recovery of sperm counts in one strain of rat, whilst proving equivocal in a different strain [55]. Protection can be achieved with just 2 weeks of GnRH agonist treatment prior to chemotherapy, as opposed to the longer treatment required for testosterone and oestrogen treatment [56].

Post-Cytotoxic Therapy. The use of GnRH agonists following irradiation or procarbazine treatment in adult rats has been shown to stimulate recovery of spermatogenesis. The use of a depot formulation of GnRH agonist in irradiated rats receiving 3.5 Gy, resulted in a 91% repopulation index in the treated animals at 10 weeks after irradiation, compared to 31% in the controls [57]. Similar results were obtained for treatment with GnRH agonists following procarbazine treatment [58]. GnRH agonists can be administered up to 15–20 weeks after irradiation and 6 weeks later differentiating germ cells derived from surviving stem cells were seen in 80 and 30% of tubules in rats receiving 3.5 [58] and 6 Gy [33], respectively. In control animals that did not receive the GnRH agonist, spermatogenesis was only restored in 10% of tubules.

Mechanism for Protection of Spermatogenesis in Rats Treated with GnRH Agonist or Sex Steroids. The fact that spermatogenesis can be restored in rats by hormonal manipulation after cytotoxic therapy suggests that the mechanism may not simply be interruption of the HPG axis to prevent germ cells from actively proliferating and protecting these 'resting' cells from being killed by the cytotoxic treatment. A study treated hpg-deficient mice, which mimic the immature or GnRH antagonist-suppressed testis, with chemotherapy and irradiation. No cytoprotective effect of being gonadotropin-deficient was demonstrated in these animals when they received chemotherapy or irradiation [59]. This study supports the view that GnRH antagonist treatment does not simply cause the germ cells to enter a resting and less sensitive state, preventing their death. Instead, it has been shown that treatment of rats with GnRH agonist, prior to procarbazine treatment, releases the germ cells from the block on differentiation that would otherwise occur [60].

Re-stimulation of spermatogonial differentiation begins 4 weeks after treatment with GnRH antagonist. It is proposed that GnRH antagonists reduce the high levels of intra-testicular testosterone caused by irradiation, leading to a reduction in both interstitial volume and testicular oedema and thus allowing resumption of spermatogenesis [34].

A recent study has attempted to identify whether the block in spermatogonial differentiation following irradiation is due to damage to germ cells or somatic cells [61]. Transplantation of irradiated immature rat germ cells into a non-irradiated rat testis resulted in spermatogenesis; however transplantation of non-irradiated, immature rat germ cells into an irradiated rat testis did not permit spermatogenesis in the donor. Spermatogenesis could be rescued in these animals by the administration of GnRH antagonists. Conversely if irradiated rat germ cells were transplanted into irradiated mouse testes (which do not exhibit a block on spermatogonial differentiation) then spermatogenesis was possible [61].

It must be noted that these studies were carried out in adult rats with established spermatogenesis. The results of these studies cannot be directly applied to immature animals because of differences in the gonadal environment that have already been discussed. Therefore studies using animal models with relevance to human childhood are required to test the effect of hormonal manipulation on the immature testis, treated with cytotoxic therapy.

Hormonal Manipulation of the Primate Testis

Attempts to recreate the effects of GnRH agonists/antagonists on radiation-induced cytotoxicity in a non-human primate have been unsuccessful [62, 63]. Adult macaques were irradiated with 6.7 Gy alone or in combination with GnRH-antagonist treatment and monitored for 18 months. A biopsy at 18 months after radiation alone revealed 3.0% of seminiferous tubule cross-sections had germ cells, whereas in those receiving GnRH antagonist 1.9% of seminiferous tubule cross-sections contained germ cells [62]. In a second study, irradiation with 4 Gy caused a drastic decrease in sperm parameters in both control and GnRH antagonist treated animals, followed by a partial recovery, which was significantly slower in the early phases of recovery in the GnRH antagonist group compared with the vehicle group [63].

Hormonal Manipulation of the Human Testis

Studies of hormonal manipulation in humans have been largely unsuccessful in preserving fertility in patients treated for cancer [for review see, 35]. The addition of a GnRH antagonist in 20 adult men treated for Hodgkin's lymphoma failed to prevent oligozoospermia during the years of follow-up. In another study of 6 men receiving GnRH agonist in addition to chemotherapy for lymphoma, only 1 of 6 recovered active spermatogenesis; however no control group was used in this study. The use of GnRH agonist prior to chemotherapy in patients with germ cell tumours led to reproductive toxicity in all patients with an identical recovery time in those receiving GnRH agonist compared with controls. Similarly recovery was seen in all patients receiving radiotherapy for seminoma regardless of whether they received GnRH agonist with cyproterone acetate or radiotherapy alone. Suppression of the HPG axis using medroxyprogesterone acetate (MPA) at the same time as cytotoxic therapy in testicular cancer patients also failed to induce recovery of sperm cell production compared to controls; however the initial FSH levels of those treated with MPA tended to be higher, which may have indicated a higher level of damage to the seminiferous epithelium of the MPA group prior to the start of treatment. Attempts to restore spermatogenesis in patients who had previously been rendered azoospermic following cancer treatment were also unsuccessful using treatment with MPA for 12 weeks. All of the men remained azoospermic with complete absence of germ cells at biopsy. Only 1 of 7 clinical trials resulted in protection of spermatogenesis. However this study was in adult patients treated with cyclophosphamide for nephritis rather than cancer. Testosterone therapy resulted in recovery by 6 months in 5 of 5 patients compared with 1 of 10 who did not receive testosterone.

Many of the human studies were carried out before it became clear that hormonal treatments in rodent studies were demonstrating restoration rather than protection of spermatogenesis, therefore failure of human studies are probably not surprising. There have been no such studies in pre-pubertal patients and further studies on the immature testis are required. As attempts to restore spermatogenesis with GnRH suppression in humans have thus far failed to preserve or rescue fertility, such techniques are not currently considered an effective treatment option.

Germ Cell Transplantation and Testis Tissue Xenografts

Removal of testicular material from the patient before cytotoxic treatment may potentially be used for transplant back into the patient (autotransplantation) once the treatment has been completed, or alternatively this material could be transplanted into a host of a different species (xenotransplantation) to undergo spermatogenesis (fig. 9). Mature germ cells produced by these techniques could, if appropriate, be used for ARTs such as intra-cytoplasmic sperm injection (ICSI).

Germ Cell Transplantation

Full spermatogenesis has been achieved in rodents using spermatogonial transplantation [64]. In this study spermatogonia, including the stem cell population were isolated from donor mice. The cell suspension was then transferred into the seminiferous tubules of recipient mice using a micro-injection technique. The animals were maintained for between 48 and 230 days before being killed. Spermatogenesis was demonstrated with both donor and endogenous germ cells at all stages, including the presence of mature spermatozoa. In addition the use of this technique produced spermatozoa that were capable of fertilization and production of progeny. Complete spermatogenesis has also been achieved with transplants of spermatogonial stem cells from rats or hamsters into a mouse host [65, 66]. Attempts to graft cells from more distant species such as rabbits, dogs, large domestic animals [67] and baboons [68] into a mouse host often result in colonisation, but these cells usually fail to differentiate beyond spermatogonia.

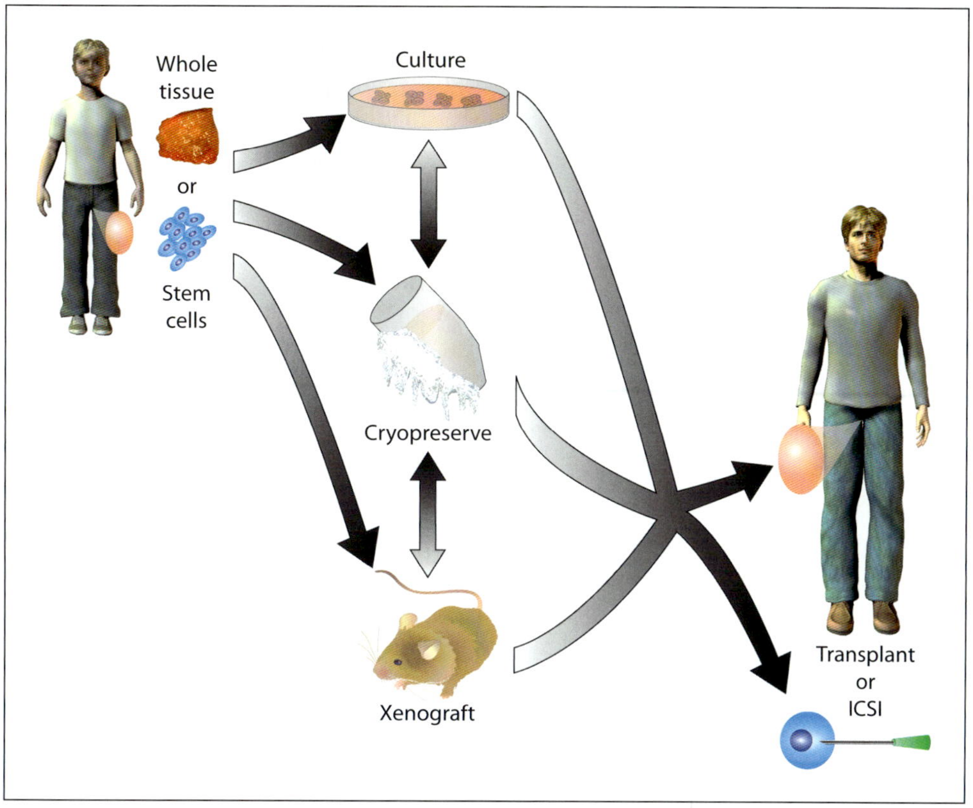

Fig. 9. Potential strategies for fertility preservation in young males prior to cytotoxic therapy. Germline stem cells or whole testicular tissue may be removed from the testis prior to cancer treatment. This material may be cryopreserved, cultured or xenografted. The material may be replaced in the host testis following the completion of treatment or alternatively mature germ cells may be recovered and used for assisted reproduction (ICSI).

Attempts to xenotransplant human spermatogonial stem cells into mice resulted in no donor germ cells surviving [69]. This experiment was performed in mice that were aspermatogenic due to lack of a normal c-kit receptor (W/W^v mutants) and also in SCID mice treated with busulphan to kill endogenous germ cells, prior to grafting. In addition the use of a GnRH agonist did not enhance spermatogenic recovery in mice treated with busulphan prior to grafting [69]. The experiment involved an anti-proacrosin antibody to detect donor germ cells and this may have prevented the identification of less differentiated germ cells if they were present. A second study demonstrated the survival of human spermatogonial stem cells in the seminiferous tubules of a mouse host for at least 6 months. Proliferation occurred but these cells did not differentiate [70]. There has been a single report describing full spermatogenesis and the production of spermatozoa in approximately 25% of mice receiving human spermatogonia [71], but despite this promising report no further reports have emerged from this group and no other group has reproduced these results and therefore these results require further confirmation.

A possible explanation for the failure of spermatogonial stem cells to develop in xenotransplant studies may be the lack of a compatible niche in the mouse host testis capable of supporting germ cells from distant species. The importance of the supporting somatic cells in recipients has already been discussed in the context of the block on differentiation caused by cytotoxic therapy [61]. The interaction between Sertoli cells and germ cells is important for establishing germ cell differentiation and spermatogenesis. This includes the production of stem cell factor from Sertoli cells, which interacts with its receptor c-kit, on the germ cell membrane. In the mouse a mutation in the gene encoding stem cell factor results in a failure of spermatogonial differentiation [72]. However differentiation of spermatogonia can resume when germ cells are transplanted from a mutant mouse into the seminiferous tubules of another mouse that does not have the mutation [73]. These studies support a hypothesis that the success of germ cell transplantation between species requires compatible host Sertoli cells, which form part of the niche that can support the donor germ cells.

Autotransplantation of human germ cells has been attempted in a study using single cell suspensions that had been removed and cryopreserved prior to cancer treatment in 11 adult men. The material was re-introduced into the testes of the donor following the completion of treatment in 5 cases. Unfortunately the results of this study have not yet been published [74].

Selection of normal germ cells for autotransplantation is important to avoid the risk of re-introducing cancer to the patient, which is known to occur in a mouse model [75]. In addition selection of spermatogonial stem cells may also improve efficiency of seminiferous tubule colonisation, as only 2 of every 10^4 germ cells is a spermatogonial stem cell [76]. Selection and enrichment of mouse spermatogonial stem cells may be achieved by fluorescence-activated cell sorting using antibodies directed against cell surface proteins such as c-kit, and α6 integrin. This technique can enrich the spermatogonial stem cell population 166-fold in a cryptorchid mouse model [77] and it may be possible to use similar methods to select human spermatogonial stem cells, providing specific cell surface markers can be identified.

Transplantation of Stem Cells from Other Lineages

In addition to transplantation of germ cells, a recent publication claimed that GFP-positive bone marrow stem cells, injected into the seminiferous tubules of busulphan-treated mice were able to undergo differentiation to germ cell and somatic cell lineages [78]. However this did not occur in a similar experiment in which the recipient was a W/W^{v} mouse. The germ cell differentiation seen in the busulphan-treated animals did not progress beyond spermatocytes. Where donor cells differentiated, there tended to be some endogenous recovering germ cells and it has been postulated that they induce the transdifferentiation of these bone marrow cells [78]. Further studies are required before we can assume that stem cells from adult tissues may be used to re-establish the germ cell population.

Testis Tissue Xenografting

The concept of testis tissue grafting to restore fertility has existed for many years. Tissue may be removed from the donor and transplanted subcutaneously, directly into the testis or beneath the kidney capsule in a host animal. Studies thus far have used immunodeficient mouse strains as recipients for these techniques.

Transplantation of whole testis tissue, which will contain both germ cells and the supporting cells, would overcome the problem of lack of compatible supporting Sertoli cells, in addition to avoiding the technical difficulties of injecting germ cells into the testis. Xenografting of testis tissue has been successful in several species and supported full spermatogenesis when mice received subcutaneous grafts from newborn mice, pigs, goats and rhesus monkeys [79]. Grafting of immature mouse testis tissue into a recipient mouse has been shown to produce full spermatogenesis and production of spermatozoa [80], whereas grafting of adult tissue was not successful. It is unclear why this is the case but may be related to the ability of immature tissue to survive relative ischaemia or demonstrate more efficient angiogenesis than adult donor tissue [80]. Another problem, which may be encountered with ectopic grafting, is fluid accumulation in the tubular lumen and subsequent atrophy [81]. This occurs more readily with mouse grafts and was much less likely with non-rodent donors.

Despite the success of grafting tissue from many species, there are also species in which full spermatogenesis does not occur. In grafts of bovine and equine tissue, spermatogenesis arrested in most cases at meiosis [82]. The marmoset is another species in which full spermatogenesis has not been demonstrated, with failure to develop beyond the spermatogonial stage [83]. This was associated with low androgen levels produced by the graft in the castrated host. In an attempt to overcome this problem, further experiments were performed using co-grafting of hamster testicular tissue, which is known to produce androgen in the host. However this did not result in germ cell differentiation [83]. An important difference between the marmoset and the human is the absence of exon 10 from the marmoset LH receptor gene [84]. This means that the receptor does not respond to LH, but instead a chorionic gonadotropin-like molecule is produced, which can activate the receptor. In view of this an attempt was made to modify the marmoset grafting experiment with administration of hCG; however this did not improve the result [85]. When testis tissue was grafted autologously into newborn marmosets, germ cells begin meiosis but arrest at the primary spermatocyte stage. Suggested reasons for failure to differentiate further include hyperthermia due to ectopic position of the graft, insufficient testosterone secretion or inadequate structural organisation of the seminiferous epithelium [86].

Although xenografting has failed to produce mature germ cells in the marmoset, it has been successful in a different primate model. Transplantation of immature testis tissue from 13-month-old rhesus monkeys, subcutaneously onto the back of ICR/SCID mice, resulted in accelerated spermatogenesis with production of mature sperm within 7 months, whereas the testes of controls remained undeveloped at 24 months [79]. Furthermore, 80% of the spermatozoa generated from donor tissue appeared viable and ICSI resulted in 3 of 16 injected oocytes developing to the blastocyst stage. The testis grafts were also able to produce testosterone as evidenced by the increase in seminal vesicle size in the host animal, despite castration prior to grafting [79].

This phenomenon of accelerated spermatogenesis had already been demonstrated in grafts from several species [79], but is particularly important as some of the donor species (i.e. rhesus monkeys) [79] do not naturally reach full spermatogenesis until 4 years of age, which is greater than the lifespan of a potential recipient mouse. Therefore with accelerated development, grafts from primates can develop full spermatogenesis within the lifetime of a rodent host.

Grafting of human tissue was first reported over 30 years ago [87]. This study involved the grafting of fetal human tissue subcutaneously into the lateral abdominal wall of nude mice. The resulting grafts were excised and examined 4–8 weeks later. They had become richly vascularised and contained seminiferous tubules with recognisable gonocytes and undifferentiated Sertoli cells. Subsequent studies of human testis grafting have only recently been reported [80, 88, 89]. These studies involved the grafting of human testis tissue into mouse hosts. Subcutaneous grafting of human adult testis tissue failed to result in the establishment of spermatogenesis within the graft and most of the grafts developed sclerosis or were Sertoli cell only. Rare spermatogonia were seen in 21–23% of the 74 grafts [80]. In another study spermatogonial stem cell survival was occasionally seen in cases in which spermatogenesis had been suppressed with cyproterone acetate and oestrogen prior to grafting [89]. Grafting using fetal human tissue has also been attempted. This resulted in the formation of lumina within the tubules and accelerated maturation of Sertoli cells, but the germ cells present would not develop beyond spermatogonia [88]. Survival of spermatogonia was also detected in grafts taken from pre-pubertal cryptorchid testes, transplanted into the scrotum of host mice [90].

The overall success of xenografting in rodents and primates, such as the rhesus monkey, may be related to the organisation of spermatogenesis in these species.

In adulthood a single stage of spermatogenesis is seen in a cross-section of the seminiferous tubule. Species such as the marmoset and the human show multiple stages of spermatogenesis within tubular cross-sections and this difference may explain why the xenografting experiments to not produce spermatozoa in these species [86].

In Vitro Germ Cell Differentiation

An alternative approach to differentiating germ cells in host animals could involve in vitro germ cell differentiation. In a study of men with pre-meiotic maturation arrest, primary spermatocytes have been reported to differentiate in vitro to produce spermatids, which were subsequently used for successful intracytoplasmic injection and resulted in the birth of a normal baby [91].

A recent study has investigated in vitro culture of human germ stem cell-like cells, which were able to proliferate and express germ stem cell markers [92]. These cells differentiated in culture under certain conditions and expressed germ cell markers, although they did not produce sperm-like cells. Furthermore, injection of spermatid-like cells into oocytes resulted in activation of the oocyte, but did not result in implantation when transferred to the uteri of the patients spouse [92].

Cryopreservation of Tissue

For any of the techniques described above to be successful an appropriate method of preservation of cells or tissue is required, particularly if the specimen is going to be stored for long periods prior to grafting. Successful cryopreservation of spermatogonial stem cells [66] and testis tissue [93] has been achieved in many species including mice, pigs and goats prior to grafting into mouse hosts [93]. These experiments resulted in the generation of fertile donor spermatozoa.

A study of testis tissue cryopreservation prior to grafting in immature rhesus monkeys has demonstrated the importance of choosing the appropriate cryoprotectant. Without cryoprotectant none of the testis tissue grafts survive following transplantation into mice and there is variation in the effectiveness of different cryoprotectants in different circumstances [94]. Survival of tissue can be achieved without using a controlled cooling method described for previous studies [94]. Prior to cryopreservation it is potentially important to be able to store cooled tissue for short periods of time, if cryobanks are to be established. Immature rhesus monkey grafts can be stored in ice-cold medium for 24 h without any adverse effects on graft survival or initiation of spermatogenesis. This would allow samples to be taken during office hours and transported to a central bank prior to cryopreservation [94].

Assisted Reproductive Techniques

Many of the above techniques could result in the production of germ cells in the later stages of spermatogenesis; however in many cases the yield may be low and ARTs will be required to produce progeny.

Spermatozoa taken from cryopreserved testis tissue have been used for ICSI and resulted in successful pregnancy [95]. As ICSI does not require the functions of spermatozoa such as motility or oocyte penetration, attempts to perform the technique have also been successful when less differentiated cell types are used, including elongate spermatids and even round spermatids [for review see, 96], and one group even reported success with intracytoplasmic injection of secondary spermatocytes, a result which has not been further confirmed by the same or another group [97]. The use of cryopreserved immature germ cells for ARTs in adulthood would be ideal for use in patients treated for cancer in childhood, who lacked mature germ cell types when their treatment commenced.

A Word of Caution

Despite the advances in experimental techniques to preserve and restore male fertility, there are many aspects that require caution. It is important to ensure that the use of these techniques does not result in harm to the patient or any resulting progeny.

When considering the potential application of grafting techniques, potential dangers must be evaluated, such as re-introduction of tumour into the patient from the graft. This has been demonstrated in rats, where introduction of as little as 20 leukaemic cells mixed with germ cells was enough to cause cancer relapse in 3 of 5 animals [75]. Fluorescence-activated cell sorting of spermatogonial stem cells from leukaemic mice and transplantation into recipient mice can prevent re-introduction of leukaemia [98]. In addition to re-introducing tumour, there are also theoretical risks of transmission of viruses or prions, DNA damage, congenital abnormalities and abnormal imprinting [99].

The use of ARTs must also be considered with caution. ICSI itself has been associated with an increased risk of chromosomal abnormality and birth defects [96]. A recent study has also shown that boys conceived by ICSI have a significant reduction in testosterone and a raised LH:testosterone ratio when compared to naturally conceived boys at 3 months postnatal age [100]. However all these effects may be related to the underlying cause of sub-fertility on the paternal side rather than a direct effect of ICSI itself. There are also theoretical risks of malformation and imprinting defects in the offspring of patients when immature cell types are used for intracytoplasmic injection [96].

The use of germ cells taken from children who are being treated or have previously been treated for cancer may add further complication for their use in ARTs. DNA damage in gametes has been suggested as a potential consequence of cancer or its treatment; however a study of men who had been treated for cancer in childhood showed that their sperm carried as much healthy DNA as controls [17]. Therefore DNA damage and congenital abnormalities as well as abnormal imprinting are theoretical but as yet unproven potential dangers for the offspring of male patients treated for childhood cancer [99].

Conclusions

In the long term, infertility is an important potential consequence of treatment for cancer in childhood. Although the risks may be minimised by advances in cancer treatment regimens, it is likely that there will remain a proportion of patients for whom strategies to preserve fertility are required. Identification of patients at significant risk of infertility is important, particularly as the condition does not manifest until after the onset of puberty. These patients should be offered established methods of fertility preservation, such as semen cryopreservation, where applicable. In pre-pubertal patients further research is required to develop strategies that will allow the future production of mature germ cells and therefore preserve fertility in these patients.

Understanding the mechanism of gonadal damage is important for developing techniques to preserve fertility. These mechanisms appear to differ between species and this is reflected in the differing results of fertility preservation strategies between rodents and primates, particularly with regard to hormonal manipulation of the gonadal environment. Translation of successful hormonal manipulation studies from the rodent into primates, including the human, has been unsuccessful. Primate models, such as the marmoset, which show many similarities to the human in terms of male gonadal development, may be invaluable for studies that involve manipulation of the gonadal environment.

There have been major advances in testicular transplantation studies in animal models. Immature testis tissue from many species can be grafted into mice to produce donor sperm. Further research is required to translate these studies into success with human testis tissue grafts. These studies, in conjunction with established techniques for assisted reproduction, offer some hope for the future fertility of childhood cancer survivors.

Acknowledgements

We would like to thank Ted Pinner for his assistance with the illustrations.

References

1 Anderson RA, Sharpe RM: Regulation of inhibin production in the human male and its clinical applications. Int J Androl 2000;23:136–144.
2 Anderson RA, Fulton N, Cowan G, Coutts S, Saunders PT: Conserved and divergent patterns of expression of DAZL, VASA and OCT4 in the germ cells of the human fetal ovary and testis. BMC Dev Biol 2007;7:136.
3 Gaskell TL, Esnal A, Robinson LL, Anderson RA, Saunders PT: Immunohistochemical profiling of germ cells within the human fetal testis: identification of three subpopulations. Biol Reprod 2004;71:2012–2021.
4 Pauls K, Schorle H, Jeske W, et al: Spatial expression of germ cell markers during maturation of human fetal male gonads: an immunohistochemical study. Hum Reprod 2006;21:397–404.
5 Castrillon DH, Quade BJ, Wang TY, Quigley C, Crum CP: The human VASA gene is specifically expressed in the germ cell lineage. Proc Natl Acad Sci USA 2000;97:9585–9590.
6 Mann DR, Fraser HM: The neonatal period: a critical interval in male primate development. J Endocrinol 1996;149:191–197.
7 Wu FC, Butler GE, Kelnar CJ, Huhtaniemi I, Veldhuis JD: Ontogeny of pulsatile gonadotropin releasing hormone secretion from midchildhood, through puberty, to adulthood in the human male: a study using deconvolution analysis and an ultrasensitive immunofluorometric assay. J Clin Endocrinol Metab 1996;81:1798–1805.
8 Chemes HE: Infancy is not a quiescent period of testicular development. Int J Androl 2001;24:2–7.
9 Kelnar CJ, McKinnell C, Walker M, et al: Testicular changes during infantile 'quiescence' in the marmoset and their gonadotrophin dependence: a model for investigating susceptibility of the prepubertal human testis to cancer therapy? Hum Reprod 2002;17:1367–1378.
10 Berensztein EB, Sciara MI, Rivarola MA, Belgorosky A: Apoptosis and proliferation of human testicular somatic and germ cells during prepuberty: high rate of testicular growth in newborns mediated by decreased apoptosis. J Clin Endocrinol Metab 2002;87:5113–5118.
11 Ferrara D, Hallmark N, Scott H, et al: Acute and long-term effects of in utero exposure of rats to di(n-butyl) phthalate on testicular germ cell development and proliferation. Endocrinology 2006;147:5352–5362.
12 Jahnukainen K, Ehmcke J, Soder O, Schlatt S: Clinical potential and putative risks of fertility preservation in children utilizing gonadal tissue or germline stem cells. Pediatr Res 2006;59:40R–47R.
13 van der Meer Y, Huiskamp R, Davids JA, van der Tweel I, de Rooij DG: The sensitivity to X rays of mouse spermatogonia that are committed to differentiate and of differentiating spermatogonia. Radiat Res 1992;130:296–302.
14 Sharpe. RM: Regulation of Spermatogenesis; in Knobil E, Neill JD (eds): The Physiology of Reproduction. New York, Raven Press, 1994, pp 1363–1434.
15 Clermont Y: The cycle of the seminiferous epithelium in man. Am J Anat 1963;112:35–51.
16 Millar MR, Sharpe RM, Weinbauer GF, Fraser HM, Saunders PT: Marmoset spermatogenesis: organizational similarities to the human. Int J Androl 2000;23:266–277.
17 Thomson AB, Campbell AJ, Irvine DC, Anderson RA, Kelnar CJ, Wallace WH: Semen quality and spermatozoal DNA integrity in survivors of childhood cancer: a case-control study. Lancet 2002;360:361–367.
18 Wallace WH, Anderson RA, Irvine DS: Fertility preservation for young patients with cancer: who is at risk and what can be offered? Lancet Oncol 2005;6:209–218.
19 Thomson AB, Critchley HO, Kelnar CJ, Wallace WH: Late reproductive sequelae following treatment of childhood cancer and options for fertility preservation. Best Pract Res Clin Endocrinol Metab 2002;16:311–334.
20 Wallace WH, Thomson AB: Preservation of fertility in children treated for cancer. Arch Dis Child 2003;88:493–496.
21 Papadakis V, Vlachopapadopoulou E, Van Syckle K, et al: Gonadal function in young patients successfully treated for Hodgkin disease. Med Pediatr Oncol 1999;32:366–372.

22 Clifton DK, Bremner WJ: The effect of testicular X-irradiation on spermatogenesis in man. A comparison with the mouse. J Androl 1983;4:387–392.
23 Rowley MJ, Leach DR, Warner GA, Heller CG: Effect of graded doses of ionizing radiation on the human testis. Radiat Res 1974;59:665–678.
24 Petersen PM, Giwercman A, Daugaard G, et al: Effect of graded testicular doses of radiotherapy in patients treated for carcinoma-in-situ in the testis. J Clin Oncol 2002;20:1537–1543.
25 Howell SJ, Shalet SM: Spermatogenesis after cancer treatment: damage and recovery. J Natl Cancer Inst Monogr 2005;34:12–17.
26 Ogilvy-Stuart AL, Clark DJ, Wallace WH, et al: Endocrine deficit after fractionated total body irradiation. Arch Dis Child 1992;67:1107–1110.
27 Socie G, Salooja N, Cohen A, et al: Nonmalignant late effects after allogeneic stem cell transplantation. Blood 2003;101:3373–3385.
28 Wallace WH, Shalet SM, Lendon M, Morris-Jones PH: Male fertility in long-term survivors of childhood acute lymphoblastic leukaemia. Int J Androl 1991;14:312–319.
29 Wallace WH, Shalet SM, Crowne EC, Morris-Jones PH, Gattamaneni HR, Price DA: Gonadal dysfunction due to cis-platinum. Med Pediatr Oncol 1989;17:409–413.
30 Meistrich ML, Wilson G, Brown BW, da Cunha MF, Lipshultz LI: Impact of cyclophosphamide on long-term reduction in sperm count in men treated with combination chemotherapy for Ewing and soft tissue sarcomas. Cancer 1992;70:2703–2712.
31 Pont J, Albrecht W: Fertility after chemotherapy for testicular germ cell cancer. Fertil Steril 1997;68:1–5.
32 Schrader M, Muller M, Straub B, Miller K: The impact of chemotherapy on male fertility: a survey of the biologic basis and clinical aspects. Reprod Toxicol 2001;15:611–617.
33 Shuttlesworth GA, de Rooij DG, Huhtaniemi I, et al: Enhancement of A spermatogonial proliferation and differentiation in irradiated rats by gonadotropin-releasing hormone antagonist administration. Endocrinology 2000;141:37–49.
34 Porter KL, Shetty G, Meistrich ML: Testicular edema is associated with spermatogonial arrest in irradiated rats. Endocrinology 2006;147:1297–1305.
35 Shetty G, Meistrich ML: Hormonal approaches to preservation and restoration of male fertility after cancer treatment. J Natl Cancer Inst Monogr 2005;34:36–39.
36 Jahnukainen K, Ehmcke J, Nurmio M, Schlatt S: Irradiation causes acute and long-term spermatogonial depletion in cultured and xenotransplanted testicular tissue from juvenile nonhuman primates. Endocrinology 2007;148:5541–5548.
37 van Alphen MM, van de Kant HJ, de Rooij DG: Depletion of the spermatogonia from the seminiferous epithelium of the rhesus monkey after X irradiation. Radiat Res 1988;113:473–486.
38 van Alphen MM, van de Kant HJ, de Rooij DG: Repopulation of the seminiferous epithelium of the rhesus monkey after X irradiation. Radiat Res 1988;113:487–500.
39 de Rooij DG, van de Kant HJ, Dol R, et al: Long-term effects of irradiation before adulthood on reproductive function in the male rhesus monkey. Biol Reprod 2002;66:486–494.
40 Darzy KH, Shalet SM: Hypopituitarism after cranial irradiation. J Endocrinol Invest 2005;28(suppl):78–87.
41 Rappaport R, Brauner R, Czernichow P, et al: Effect of hypothalamic and pituitary irradiation on pubertal development in children with cranial tumors. J Clin Endocrinol Metab 1982;54:1164–1168.
42 Constine LS, Woolf PD, Cann D, et al: Hypothalamic-pituitary dysfunction after radiation for brain tumors. N Engl J Med 1993;328:87–94.
43 Ogilvy-Stuart AL, Stirling HF, Kelnar CJ, et al: Treatment of radiation-induced growth hormone deficiency with growth hormone-releasing hormone. Clin Endocrinol 1997;46:571–578.
44 Rueffer U, Breuer K, Josting A, et al: Male gonadal dysfunction in patients with Hodgkin's disease prior to treatment. Ann Oncol 2001;12:1307–1311.
45 Petersen PM, Giwercman A, Skakkebaek NE, Rorth M: Gonadal function in men with testicular cancer. Semin Oncol 1998;25:224–233.
46 van der Kaaij MA, Heutte N, Le Stang N, et al: Gonadal function in males after chemotherapy for early-stage Hodgkin's lymphoma treated in four subsequent trials by the European Organisation for Research and Treatment of Cancer: EORTC Lymphoma Group and the Groupe d'Etude des Lymphomes de l'Adulte. J Clin Oncol 2007;25:2825–2832.
47 Viviani S, Santoro A, Ragni G, Bonfante V, Bestetti O, Bonadonna G: Gonadal toxicity after combination chemotherapy for Hodgkin's disease. Comparative results of MOPP vs ABVD. Eur J Cancer Clin Oncol 1985;21:601–605.

48 Hovav Y, Dan-Goor M, Yaffe H, Almagor M: Electroejaculation before chemotherapy in adolescents and young men with cancer. Fertil Steril 2001;75:811–813.

49 Schover LR, Brey K, Lichtin A, Lipshultz LI, Jeha S: Oncologists' attitudes and practices regarding banking sperm before cancer treatment. J Clin Oncol 2002;20:1890–1897.

50 Schover LR, Brey K, Lichtin A, Lipshultz LI, Jeha S: Knowledge and experience regarding cancer, infertility, and sperm banking in younger male survivors. J Clin Oncol 2002;20:1880–1889.

51 Edge B, Holmes D, Makin G: Sperm banking in adolescent cancer patients. Arch Dis Child 2006; 91:149–152.

52 Blackhall FH, Atkinson AD, Maaya MB, et al: Semen cryopreservation, utilisation and reproductive outcome in men treated for Hodgkin's disease. Br J Cancer 2002;87:381–384.

53 Kurdoglu B, Wilson G, Parchuri N, Ye WS, Meistrich ML: Protection from radiation-induced damage to spermatogenesis by hormone treatment. Radiat Res 1994;139:97–102.

54 Parchuri N, Wilson G, Meistrich ML: Protection by gonadal steroid hormones against procarbazine-induced damage to spermatogenic function in LBNF1 hybrid rats. J Androl 1993;14:257–266.

55 Ward JA, Robinson J, Furr BJ, Shalet SM, Morris ID: Protection of spermatogenesis in rats from the cytotoxic procarbazine by the depot formulation of Zoladex, a gonadotropin-releasing hormone agonist. Cancer Res 1990;50:568–574.

56 Kangasniemi M, Wilson G, Parchuri N, Huhtaniemi I, Meistrich ML: Rapid protection of rat spermatogenic stem cells against procarbazine by treatment with a gonadotropin-releasing hormone antagonist (Nal-Glu) and an antiandrogen (flutamide). Endocrinology 1995;136:2881–2888.

57 Meistrich ML, Kangasniemi M: Hormone treatment after irradiation stimulates recovery of rat spermatogenesis from surviving spermatogonia. J Androl 1997;18:80–87.

58 Meistrich ML, Wilson G, Huhtaniemi I: Hormonal treatment after cytotoxic therapy stimulates recovery of spermatogenesis. Cancer Res 1999;59:3557–3560.

59 Crawford BA, Spaliviero JA, Simpson JM, Handelsman DJ: Testing the gonadal regression-cytoprotection hypothesis. Cancer Res 1998;58: 5105–5109.

60 Meistrich ML, Wilson G, Kangasniemi M, Huhtaniemi I: Mechanism of protection of rat spermatogenesis by hormonal pretreatment: stimulation of spermatogonial differentiation after irradiation. J Androl 2000;21:464–469.

61 Zhang Z, Shao S, Meistrich ML: The radiation-induced block in spermatogonial differentiation is due to damage to the somatic environment, not the germ cells. J Cell Physiol 2007;211:149–158.

62 Boekelheide K, Schoenfeld HA, Hall SJ, et al: Gonadotropin-releasing hormone antagonist (Cetrorelix) therapy fails to protect nonhuman primates *(Macaca arctoides)* from radiation-induced spermatogenic failure. J Androl 2005;26: 222–234.

63 Kamischke A, Kuhlmann M, Weinbauer GF, et al: Gonadal protection from radiation by GnRH antagonist or recombinant human FSH: a controlled trial in a male nonhuman primate *(Macaca fascicularis)*. J Endocrinol 2003;179:183–194.

64 Brinster RL, Avarbock MR: Germline transmission of donor haplotype following spermatogonial transplantation. Proc Natl Acad Sci USA 1994;91:11303–11307.

65 Clouthier DE, Avarbock MR, Maika SD, Hammer RE, Brinster RL: Rat spermatogenesis in mouse testis. Nature 1996;381:418–421.

66 Ogawa T, Dobrinski I, Avarbock MR, Brinster RL: Xenogeneic spermatogenesis following transplantation of hamster germ cells to mouse testes. Biol Reprod 1999;60:515–521.

67 Dobrinski I, Avarbock MR, Brinster RL: Germ cell transplantation from large domestic animals into mouse testes. Mol Reprod Dev 2000;57:270–279.

68 Nagano M, McCarrey JR, Brinster RL: Primate spermatogonial stem cells colonize mouse testes. Biol Reprod 2001;64:1409–1416.

69 Reis MM, Tsai MC, Schlegel PN, et al: Xenogeneic transplantation of human spermatogonia. Zygote 2000;8:97–105.

70 Nagano M, Patrizio P, Brinster RL: Long-term survival of human spermatogonial stem cells in mouse testes. Fertil Steril 2002;78:1225–1233.

71 Sofikitis N: Transplantation of human spermatogonia into the seminiferous tubules (STs) of animal testicles results in the completion of the human meiosis and the generation of human motile spermatozoa. Fertil Steril 1999;72(suppl 1): S83–S84.

72 Brannan CI, Bedell MA, Resnick JL, et al: Developmental abnormalities in Steel17H mice result from a splicing defect in the steel factor cytoplasmic tail. Genes Dev 1992;6:1832–1842.
73 Ohta H, Yomogida K, Dohmae K, Nishimune Y: Regulation of proliferation and differentiation in spermatogonial stem cells: the role of c-kit and its ligand SCF. Development 2000;127:2125–2131.
74 Radford J, Shalet S, Lieberman B: Fertility after treatment for cancer. Questions remain over ways of preserving ovarian and testicular tissue. BMJ 1999;319:935–936.
75 Jahnukainen K, Hou M, Petersen C, Setchell B, Soder O: Intratesticular transplantation of testicular cells from leukemic rats causes transmission of leukemia. Cancer Res 2001;61:706–710.
76 Tegelenbosch RA, de Rooij DG: A quantitative study of spermatogonial multiplication and stem cell renewal in the C3H/101 F1 hybrid mouse. Mutat Res 1993;290:193–200.
77 Shinohara T, Orwig KE, Avarbock MR, Brinster RL: Spermatogonial stem cell enrichment by multiparameter selection of mouse testis cells. Proc Natl Acad Sci USA 2000;97:8346–8351.
78 Lue Y, Erkkila K, Liu PY, et al: Fate of bone marrow stem cells transplanted into the testis: potential implication for men with testicular failure. Am J Pathol 2007;170:899–908.
79 Honaramooz A, Li MW, Penedo MC, Meyers S, Dobrinski I: Accelerated maturation of primate testis by xenografting into mice. Biol Reprod 2004;70:1500–1503.
80 Geens M, De Block G, Goossens E, Frederickx V, Van Steirteghem A, Tournaye H: Spermatogonial survival after grafting human testicular tissue to immunodeficient mice. Hum Reprod 2006;21:390–396.
81 Schlatt S, Honaramooz A, Boiani M, Scholer HR, Dobrinski I: Progeny from sperm obtained after ectopic grafting of neonatal mouse testes. Biol Reprod 2003;68:2331–2335.
82 Rathi R, Honaramooz A, Zeng W, Turner R, Dobrinski I: Germ cell development in equine testis tissue xenografted into mice. Reproduction 2006;131:1091–1098.
83 Schlatt S, Kim SS, Gosden R: Spermatogenesis and steroidogenesis in mouse, hamster and monkey testicular tissue after cryopreservation and heterotopic grafting to castrated hosts. Reproduction 2002;124:339–346.
84 Gromoll J, Eiholzer U, Nieschlag E, Simoni M: Male hypogonadism caused by homozygous deletion of exon 10 of the luteinizing hormone (LH) receptor: differential action of human chorionic gonadotropin and LH. J Clin Endocrinol Metab 2000;85:2281–2286.
85 Wistuba J, Mundry M, Luetjens CM, Schlatt S: Cografting of hamster *(Phodopus sungorus)* and marmoset *(Callithrix jacchus)* testicular tissues into nude mice does not overcome blockade of early spermatogenic differentiation in primate grafts. Biol Reprod 2004;71:2087–2091.
86 Wistuba J, Luetjens CM, Wesselmann R, Nieschlag E, Simoni M, Schlatt S: Meiosis in autologous ectopic transplants of immature testicular tissue grafted to *Callithrix jacchus*. Biol Reprod 2006;74:706–713.
87 Povlsen CO, Skakkebaek NE, Rygaard J, Jensen G: Heterotransplantation of human foetal organs to the mouse mutant nude. Nature 1974;248:247–249.
88 Yu J, Cai ZM, Wan HJ, et al: Development of neonatal mouse and fetal human testicular tissue as ectopic grafts in immunodeficient mice. Asian J Androl 2006;8:393–403.
89 Schlatt S, Honaramooz A, Ehmcke J, et al: Limited survival of adult human testicular tissue as ectopic xenograft. Hum Reprod 2006;21:384–389.
90 Wyns C, Curaba M, Martinez-Madrid B, Van Langendonckt A, Francois-Xavier W, Donnez J: Spermatogonial survival after cryopreservation and short-term orthotopic immature human cryptorchid testicular tissue grafting to immunodeficient mice. Hum Reprod 2007;22:1603–1611.
91 Tesarik J, Bahceci M, Ozcan C, Greco E, Mendoza C: Restoration of fertility by in-vitro spermatogenesis. Lancet 1999;353:555–556.
92 Lee DR, Kim KS, Yang YH, et al: Isolation of male germ stem cell-like cells from testicular tissue of non-obstructive azoospermic patients and differentiation into haploid male germ cells in vitro. Hum Reprod 2006;21:471–476.
93 Honaramooz A, Snedaker A, Boiani M, Scholer H, Dobrinski I, Schlatt S: Sperm from neonatal mammalian testes grafted in mice. Nature 2002;418:778–781.
94 Jahnukainen K, Ehmcke J, Hergenrother SD, Schlatt S: Effect of cold storage and cryopreservation of immature non-human primate testicular tissue on spermatogonial stem cell potential in xenografts. Hum Reprod 2007;22:1060–1067.

95 Hovatta O, Foudila T, Siegberg R, Johansson K, von Smitten K, Reima I: Pregnancy resulting from intracytoplasmic injection of spermatozoa from a frozen-thawed testicular biopsy specimen. Hum Reprod 1996;11:2472–2473.
96 Tesarik J, Mendoza C: Using the male gamete for assisted reproduction: past, present, and future. J Androl 2003;24:317–328.
97 Sofikitis N, Mantzavinos T, Loutradis D, Yamamoto Y, Tarlatzis V, Miyagawa I: Ooplasmic injections of secondary spermatocytes for non-obstructive azoospermia. Lancet 1998;351: 1177–1178.
98 Fujita K, Ohta H, Tsujimura A, et al: Transplantation of spermatogonial stem cells isolated from leukemic mice restores fertility without inducing leukemia. J Clin Invest 2005;115:1855–1861.
99 Tournaye H, Goossens E, Verheyen G, et al: Preserving the reproductive potential of men and boys with cancer: current concepts and future prospects. Hum Reprod Update 2004;10:525–532.
100 Mau Kai C, Main KM, Andersen AN, Loft A, Skakkebaek NE, Juul A: Reduced serum testosterone levels in infant boys conceived by intracytoplasmic sperm injection. J Clin Endocrinol Metab 2007;92:2598–2603.

W. Hamish B. Wallace, MD, FRCP, FRCPCH
Royal Hospital for Sick Children, University of Edinburgh
17 Millerfield Place
Edinburgh EH9 1LW (UK)
Tel. +44 131 536 0426, Fax +44 131 536 0430, E-Mail hamish.wallace@luht.scot.nhs.uk

Wallace WHB, Kelnar CJH (eds): Endocrinopathy after Childhood Cancer Treatment.
Endocr Dev. Basel, Karger, 2009, vol 15, pp 135–158

Fertility in Female Childhood Cancer Survivors

Marie L. De Bruin[a] · Eline van Dulmen-den Broeder[b] · Marleen H. van den Berg[b] · Cornelis B. Lambalk[c]

[a]Department of Epidemiology, Netherlands Cancer Institute; [b]Department of Paediatric Oncology/ Haematology, and [c]Division of Reproductive Medicine, Department of Obstetrics and Gynaecology, VU University Medical Centre, Amsterdam, The Netherlands

Abstract

Advances in childhood cancer treatment over the past decades have significantly improved survival, resulting in a rapidly enlarging group of childhood cancer survivors. There is much concern, however, about the effects of treatment on reproductive potential. In women there is evidence that both chemotherapy and radiotherapy may have an adverse effect on ovarian function, ovarian reserve and uterine function, clinically leading to sub-fertility, infertility, premature menopause and/or adverse pregnancy outcomes. Here we will first address normal female fertility and methods to detect decreased fertility. Hence we will focus on direct effects as well as late fertility-related adverse effects caused by chemotherapy and radiotherapy, and we will conclude with a summary of current options for fertility preservation in female childhood cancer survivors.

Normal Female Fertility

Many factors influence whether a woman can produce offspring. A tightly interwoven system, the hypothalamic-pituitary-ovarian axis, is responsible for oocyte maturation, ovulation and proliferation of the uterine lining. This axis is also involved in the onset of puberty and the development of secondary sex characteristics. A successful pregnancy, however, not only requires a fully functional hypothalamic-pituitary-ovarian axis but also a uterus, which is receptive to implantation and is capable of growing with the developing fetus to term.

At birth, the hypothalamic-pituitary axis is active for a very brief period, after which it remains quiescent until puberty begins. At puberty pulsatile bursts of gonadotropin-releasing hormone (GnRH) are produced by the hypothalamus, which

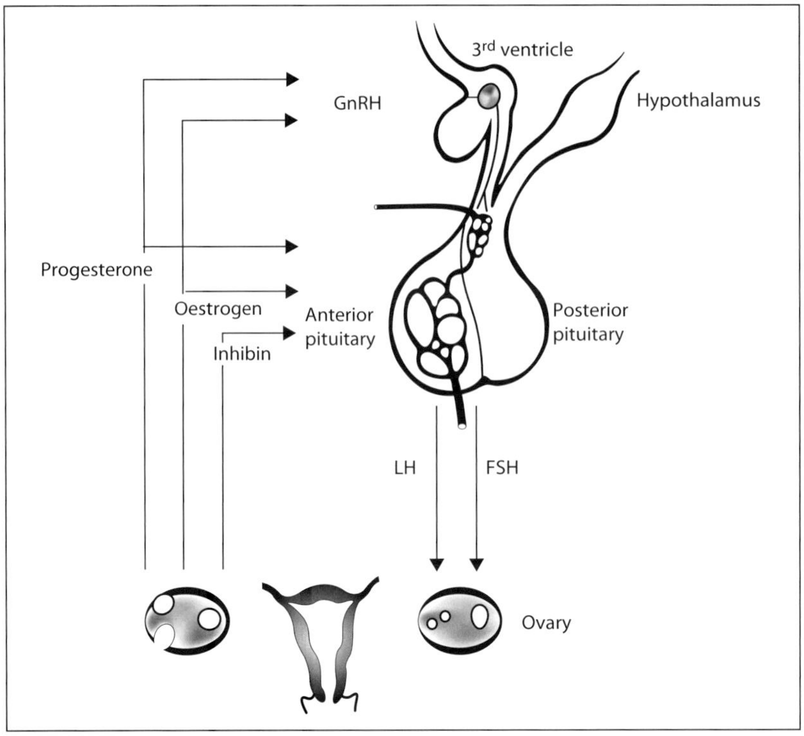

Fig. 1. The hypothalamic-pituitary-ovarian axis.

stimulate the pituitary to release follicle-stimulating hormone (FSH) and luteinising hormone (LH). These hormones, in turn, facilitate oocyte maturation in the ovaries, which results in the production of hormones involved in the development of secondary sex characteristics. On average, puberty in girls commences at the age of 11 years (standard deviation 1 year) and should progress from one Tanner stage to the next every 6–9 months. If not, one should be vigilant for gonadal damage.

In contrast to men, the number of primordial follicles in the ovaries of females is set at birth at approximately 1 million, although in recent years this view has been challenged [1]. At menarche, approximately 400,000 follicles remain, but only 300–400 will undergo further maturation in an ovulatory cycle. The ovaries are regulated by the hypothalamus and the pituitary. Their function includes oocyte maturation and ovulation, and the production of hormones.

Each month, under the influence of FSH released by the pituitary, a number of resting follicles mature to antral follicles. These maturing antral follicles produce hormones which respectively reduce FSH secretion by inhibition of the hypothalamus and the pituitary via negative feedback (inhibin B), and promote further follicle growth and the development of the endometrium (oestradiol; fig. 1).

The dominant follicle is selected from this cohort of maturing antral follicles and an LH surge, delivered by the pituitary, results in the release of the ovum from the dominant follicle into the fallopian tube. Following ovulation, the 'remains' of the dominant follicle, now called the corpus luteum, produces large amounts of progesterone involved in the development and maintenance of the uterine lining. When conception, and thus implantation, fails to occur the endometrium is shed and the menstrual cycle starts again. The number of follicles thus gradually reduces with age until approximately 1,000 follicles are left. A woman has then reached menopause at an average age of 51 years. This gradual decline of primordial follicles with age is illustrated by a model from Faddy and Gosden [2].

Any 'insult' to this tightly interwoven system may adversely affect fertility. Damage to the hypothalamic-pituitary axis may lead clinically to a delayed or arrested puberty, resulting in primary amenorrhoea if damage occurs before puberty, and secondary amenorrhoea with damage during or after puberty. Damage to the ovaries, resulting in a reduction or depletion in the primordial follicles, may lead to infertility, reduced fertility or a premature menopause with subsequent risks of menopause-related conditions. Adverse effects of treatment to the uterus may result in low birth weight babies, spontaneous abortions or miscarriages due to the inability of the uterus to carry a fetus to term.

Childhood cancer and its treatment may lead to any of the fertility defects described above [3, 4]. In general, females seem less sensitive to the adverse effects of chemotherapy than males. Studies have shown that reproductive function can usually be normal after treatment of childhood cancer. However, poor ovarian function, infertility and damage to the uterus have also been described following childhood cancer treatment [3, 4]. In addition, seemingly normal ovarian function, assessed by the resumption of regular menses after therapy, normal hormone levels, and even pregnancy, does not mean that the ovaries escaped damage. Treatment may have accelerated the decline of the non-renewable pool of primordial follicles in the ovaries, reducing fertile lifespan and resulting in premature menopause [5]. On the other hand, the absence of regular menstrual cycles does not necessarily imply infertility [3]. Mechanisms underlying recovery of ovarian function are unclear and there are no indicators that allow the identification of women who recover ovarian function, other than the fact that it is more likely to occur in younger women [6].

Detection of Decreased Fertility

General Aspects of Female Fertility Evaluation

Normal fertility requires: (1) adequate development of ovarian follicles that contain an oocyte from which preferably only one becomes dominant in readiness for ovulation; (2) ovulation; (3) normal transportation of the gametes; (4) fertilisation of the oocyte by one sperm; (5) implantation of the resulting conception, and (6) support of the conceptus such that an ongoing pregnancy results.

This highly complex constellation demands many properly functioning body features both anatomically and physiologically.

During routine evaluation of an infertile couple a number (but not all) of these functions are investigated. Briefly: (1) ovarian competence is studied; (2) anatomical conditions are evaluated that are needed to allow the gametes (oocyte and sperm) to encounter and an embryo to nidate, and (3) verification that ovulation took place and that adequate sperm is available. Moreover sexual behaviour, general health and environmental aspects need evaluation. In the context of this chapter we will briefly summarise some general features of the natural decline of fertility and practical ways by which the various sub-fertility aspects are addressed in the female [for complete reviews see, 7, 8].

Natural Decline of Female Fertility and Ovarian Reserve Testing

From studies on natural populations in which no consistent methods of birth control are applied, it has been shown that natural fertility starts to decline after the age of 30, accelerates in the mid-30s and will lead to sterility at a mean age of 41. The reduction in female fertility can also be seen in contemporary population studies. The chance of not conceiving a first child within 1 year increases from less than 5% in women in their early 20s to approximately 30% or over in the age group of 35 years and older. So although the majority of women of older age will obtain the desired pregnancy within a 1-year period, the chance of becoming sub-fertile increases approximately 6-fold in comparison with very young women. This age-related decline in fertility is the result of a progressive decrease in quality and number of oocytes from follicles left in the ovaries (ovarian reserve).

Women starting an infertility workup will undergo extensive testing. An accurate measure of the quantitative ovarian reserve would theoretically involve the counting of all follicles present in both ovaries, as was done in post-mortem studies. For obvious reasons, in ovarian reserve testing, the true size of the follicle pool has not been used as the benchmark for evaluation. Aside from its invasiveness and the potential complications of the procedure, the taking of an ovarian biopsy cannot be considered a reliable way to determine ovarian competence in an individual patient in either a quantitative or qualitative sense.

Over the past two decades a number of less invasive estimates have been proposed to predict the competence of the ovaries. Static estimates are calendar age, basal early follicular phase levels of hormones such as FSH, E_2 and inhibin B, antimullerian hormone and ultrasonic appearance of the ovary in terms of numbers of antral follicles (antral follicle count: AFC) and the volume of the ovary. Dynamic estimates are the clomiphene challenge test (CCT), the GnRH agonist stimulation test and the Exogenous FSH Ovarian Reserve Test (EFORT).

Of all these, the measurement of early follicular FSH is probably most widely used in the diagnostic workup of a couple with infertility. A raised basal FSH is associated with a decreased success rate in assisted reproduction. The number of antral follicles and ovarian volumes correlate well with female calendar ageing and can predict rather well the number of follicles that can be obtained in assisted reproductive technologies (ART). In addition, several recent studies indicate that anti-mullerian hormone could be a potential candidate for the assessment of ovarian reserve as it correlates with AFC, calendar age and ART yield. It is produced by pre-antral follicles and, as such, is a relatively stable measure of follicle numbers as a consequence of the limited inter-cyclic variability.

With regard to dynamic hormonal tests, we showed in a recent prospective study in in vitro fertilisation (IVF) patients that the best predictor of a poor response to IVF was the CCT (ROC-AUC = 0.88) while the E_2 increment in the EFORT had an ROC-AUC of 0.75 and the inhibin B-increment had an ROC-AUC of 0.86. For high response to IVF, univariate logistic regression showed that the best predictor is the inhibin B-increment in the EFORT (ROC-AUC = 0.92). The E_2 increment in the EFORT had an ROC-AUC of 0.83 which made us conclude that the EFORT is not a better predictor to identify poor responders than the CCT and that the inhibin B increment in the EFORT will best predict a high response. Others showed that GAST is a good predictor of ovarian response in ART in comparison to basal FSH and CCT.

Thus, currently available ovarian reserve tests are not sensitive and specific enough to justify general application and the ideal test has yet to be identified. Such a test in the standard diagnostic work up would potentially identify all patients with a chance of becoming pregnant and should identify poor and high responders such that it would enable us to determine for each individual patient the optimal ART stimulation scenario.

Detection of Ovulation

Regular menstrual cyclicity is usually indicative of ovulation. But ovulation needs to be confirmed. In clinical practise, detection of ovulation is based on tracing the acute changes (1) resulting from the shifting endocrine environment (detection of a rise in LH in a daily urine sample, registration of a shift in daily registered basal body temperature or the measuring of progesterone in a timed single serum sample), and (2) in anatomical appearance (disappearance/collapse of the dominant follicle and occurrence of a corpus luteum detected by means of a timed ultrasound scan).

Oligomenorrhoea and amenorrhoea are conditions in which the growth of follicles and ovulation are disturbed. These conditions contribute to about 20% of all cases of sub-fertility. According to the World Health Organisation (WHO) classification these disorders can be divided into 3 groups: WHO I, WHO II and WHO III. This classification is based on the levels of gonadotropic hormones, LH and FSH, found during laboratory testing as is routinely applied in these patients.

Class WHO I is characterised by very low levels of LH and FSH indicating disorders at the level of the brain (insufficient brain-derived GnRH) or a damaged pituitary. In WHO II patients normal LH and FSH levels are found. This class represents most (>80%) of all oligomenorrhoeic women. The most frequent disorder responsible for this is polycystic ovary syndrome which is further characterised by many small cysts in the ovaries (>12 in each) observed by ultrasound and/or signs of hyper-androgenism such as high levels of serum androgens and/or hirsutism/severe acne.

Finally WHO III patients have elevated levels of gonadotropins. This condition is present in the case of absent ovarian function which is analogous to the physiologically post-menopausal state. Indeed often these patients also report other typical menopausal complaints such as hot flushes. This latter group consists of approximately 5% of women with ovulatory disorders. However, among cancer survivors this is the most frequently encountered type of cycle disturbance.

Evaluation of the Female Reproductive Tract in Sub-Fertility

Uterus

Congenital and acquired uterine anomalies such as uterus bicornis/unicornis, septae, polyps, myomata, adhesions and adenomyosis in relation to infertility are rare and their relationship to possible sub-fertility is difficult to prove. This is even more difficult if interventions based on observed abnormalities are used in the absence of adequate published trials. Endoscopic hysteroscopy and laparoscopy, radiographic hysterosalpingography and abdominal/vaginal ultrasound are all useful techniques to determine these uterine anomalies. Reduced uterine volume and decreased elasticity of uterine musculature, which can be found in female childhood cancer survivors treated with abdominal irradiation, can be visualised by transvaginal ultrasound [9].

Assessment of Tubal Function

Tubal dysfunction with a negative impact on fertility due to disrupted transportation of the ovulated oocyte is a very important cause of sub-fertility and contributes to about 15%.

Cornerstones for evaluation of tubal function are: (1) radiographic hysterosalpingography, which visualises interior conditions and patency of the uterus and the fallopian tubes, and (2) diagnostic laparoscopy, which enables evaluation of intra-abdominal conditions that may affect fertility such as adhesions and endometriosis. Both tests are reliable, with good sensitivity and specificity profiles, so that their routine application in clinical practice is justified.

Post-Coital Test
While the fallopian tubes are important for transportation of the oocyte (and the early embryo), the cervix, with its abundantly available mucus around time of ovulation, is crucial for sperm transportation. Cervical function in this context is tested routinely with the post-coital test. Cervical disorders contribute to about 5% of sub-fertility. A well-timed post-coital test contributes significantly to models that predict the chance of pregnancy. Nevertheless its routine use in the investigation of a sub-fertile couple is questioned [8].

Effects of Cancer Treatment on Female Fertility

Decreased fertility and ovarian failure have been reported in female survivors of childhood cancer. Relative fertility rates vary according to the primary diagnosis and are linked to gonadotoxic effects of treatment [10]. It has been estimated that the biological ovarian age in childhood cancer survivors is approximately 10 years ahead of their chronological age [5].

Fertility-related adverse effects of treatment may be mediated through the hypothalamic-pituitary axis, the ovary or the uterus. Radiotherapy is known to act on all three of these systems; however, direct effects of chemotherapy on the hypothalamic-pituitary axis and the uterus have not been described.

Effect of Radiotherapy on Hypothalamic-Pituitary Axis

The hypothalamic-pituitary axis directly affects the functions of the thyroid gland, the adrenal gland and the ovaries, and can be considered the co-ordinating centre of the endocrine system. As a consequence, radiation to the hypothalamic-pituitary axis as part of treatment for childhood cancer carries a risk of inducing endocrine adverse effects. The radiation-induced damage to this axis depends on the total dose, fraction size, number of fractions and the duration [11].

Cranial (spinal) irradiation is used alone or in combination with surgery and/or chemotherapy for brain tumours and acute lymphoblastic leukaemia with central nervous system involvement, and has a damaging effect on the hypothalamic-pituitary axis. As a consequence, high-dose (>24 Gy) cranial radiotherapy is associated with a risk of delayed puberty or secondary amenorrhoea in girls, whereas lower doses, paradoxically, may result in early puberty or precocious puberty [12]. Furthermore, a recent study demonstrated that females exposed to cranial or craniospinal radiotherapy are at risk of abnormal timing of menarche [13].

Hypothalamic-pituitary dysfunction secondary to radiation is progressive over time, as there is an increase in the frequency and severity of hormonal deficits with a longer time interval after radiotherapy [11]. Several studies have investigated the late effects (i.e. effects that may manifest years after completion of cancer treatment) of radiation to the hypothalamic-pituitary axis. One study showed that the majority (64%) of girls who had received craniospinal irradiation without chemotherapy developed ovarian damage as determined by elevated gonadotropins [14]. In addition, Bath et al. [15] demonstrated that young female survivors exposed to low dose (18–24 Gy) cranial irradiation showed decreased LH secretion, an attenuated LH surge, and shorter luteal phases. Since these parameters have been associated with reduced fertility and adverse pregnancy outcomes [16, 17], monitoring this group of female survivors at regular intervals after the completion of treatment is a matter of utmost importance.

Effect of Radiotherapy on the Uterus

Uterine characteristics that may be affected by radiotherapy are: volume (growth); vascularisation, and endometrial thickness. The degree of uterine damage depends on the total radiation dose and the site of irradiation. The extent of uterine damage due to childhood radiotherapy is influenced by age. At puberty, uterine shape alters from a tubular to a pear-shaped organ with an increase in volume. Therefore, the pre-pubertal uterus is more sensitive to radiation-induced damage as uterine development is not completed before the onset of puberty.

A number of studies have investigated the direct adverse effects of irradiation on the uterus. Whole abdominal-pelvic irradiation (20–30 Gy) has been reported to result in impaired uterine development and reduced volume and vascularisation [18]. Although treatment with total body irradiation (TBI) and bone marrow transplantation involves exposure to lower doses of radiotherapy than those during abdominal irradiation, it has been demonstrated that survivors after such treatments remain at high risk of reduced uterine volume, impaired blood flow and absent endometrium [19, 20]. These abnormal uterine characteristics have been associated with adverse pregnancy outcomes such as preterm delivery and low birth weight in female childhood cancer survivors [9, 21].

Hormone replacement therapy (HRT) can improve uterine size, endometrial thickness and uterine vascularisation in female survivors [19, 22]. However, the

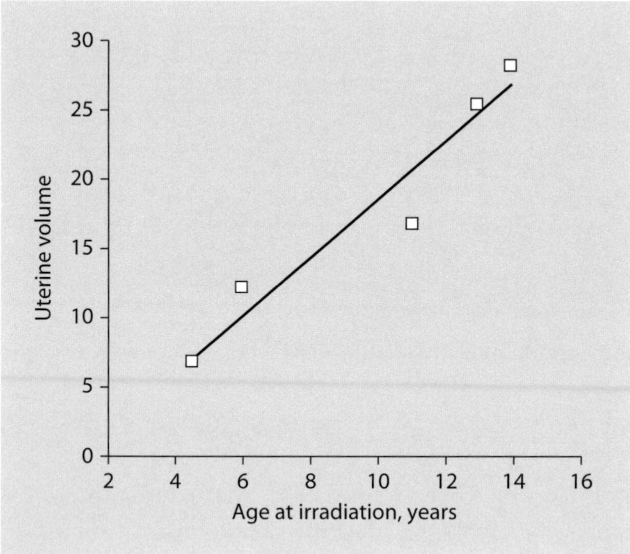

Fig. 2. Correlation between uterine volume in the 3rd month of physiological sex steroid replacement and age at irradiation ($p < 0.05$). Reprinted from Bath et al. [19], with permission from Blackwell Publishing Ltd.

appropriate dose of sex steroids is as yet unknown [20]. Furthermore, not all females may benefit to the same extent from HRT, as patients treated pre-pubertally show a significantly smaller increase in uterine volume than patients who have been irradiated after puberty. Indeed, final uterine volume after HRT showed a significant correlation with age at irradiation (fig. 2) [19].

Furthermore, high-dose radiotherapy (>30 Gy) delivered at abdominal or pelvic sites, may result in irreversible uterine damage which cannot be overcome by sex steroid replacement therapy [22, 23]. This finding is supported by the study of Larsen et al. [23] which demonstrated that in females with an apparent preserved ovarian function, with endogenous hormone production during puberty, uterine sizes can still be very small.

Effect of Treatment on the Ovaries

Treatment-induced ovarian damage may cause acute amenorrhoea during or shortly after treatment, which may be permanent or transient. Women who retain apparently normal ovarian function after treatment or regain normal ovarian function after a period of amenorrhoea (which can last months or years) still may face problems when trying to become pregnant and/or may experience premature menopause later in life (fig. 3) [6].

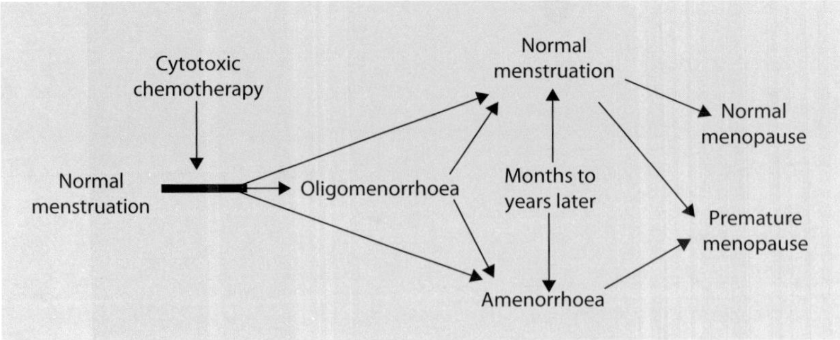

Fig. 3. The impact of chemotherapy on the menstrual cycle. Reprinted from Howell et al. [6], with permission from Elsevier.

Because many definitions of decreased fertility are used, many outcomes have been studied in childhood cancer survivors. In general, two forms of premature ovarian failure can be distinguished [24]. When ovarian failure occurs shortly after completion of therapy, it is classified as acute ovarian failure. Researchers use several cut-off points to determine acute ovarian failure rates, such as 6 or 12 months after completion of therapy, with a maximum of 5 years after cancer diagnosis.

Patients who remain (or recover) normal ovarian function during the first 5 years, may still face the risk of developing premature ovarian failure subsequently. Any occurrence of ovarian failure before age 40 is classified as premature menopause, and this may occur after the first 5 years following cancer diagnosis.

Effect of Age at Time of Treatment

Since ovarian reserve decreases with age, similar amounts of chemotherapy and/or radiotherapy may have more direct gonadotoxic effects in older compared to younger women. Taking acute ovarian failure as a measure of decreased fertility, secondary amenorrhoea rates in post-pubertal girls are higher compared to primary amenorrhoea rates in pre-pubertal girls [25]. The age effect on acute ovarian failure is also reflected in the fact that ovarian function recovery rates after bone marrow transplantation in older women are lower than in young women [26].

When premature menopause rates related to gonadotoxic treatment are compared between post- and pre-pubertal girls, however, differences are not as distinct and can even become statistically insignificant [27]. A similar age effect is seen in a cohort of 518 female survivors of Hodgkin's lymphoma treated with chemotherapy and/or supradiaphragmal radiotherapy before the age of 40 in a study by De Bruin et al. [28]: older women experience premature menopause relatively shortly after treatment, but at age 40 the cumulative incidence of premature menopause does not differ according to age. This phenomenon was also described by Haukvik et al. [29].

Regardless of the effect of decreased ovarian reserve, it has been hypothesised that post-pubertal girls may also experience more gonadotoxicity compared to pre-pubertal girls [30].

Effect of Radiotherapy

Irradiation can cause damage to immature oocytes and hasten the natural decline of the primordial follicles in the ovaries. The degree and persistence of radiation-induced damage to the ovaries depends on the age of the individual at the time of treatment, the field of radiation, the total irradiation dose, and the dose per fraction. The ovaries of younger females are more resistant to damage from irradiation. In addition, the ovaries appear to be susceptible to damage from irradiation in a dose-dependent manner [31]. Exposure to high doses of radiotherapy can cause sterility with total depletion of the primordial follicle reserve, whereas lower doses cause only partial depletion of the primordial follicle reserve, which leads to premature ovarian failure. Furthermore, it has recently been calculated that the irradiation dose required to kill 50% of the oocytes, i.e. median lethal dose, is <2 Gy [32].

Females exposed to abdominal-pelvic irradiation appear to be at highest risk of developing acute ovarian failure [25]. Radiation doses in the range of 10–30 Gy have been found to cause acute ovarian failure. However, smaller doses of radiotherapy to the ovaries are also capable of inducing this phenomenon [25]. Furthermore, conditioning regimens given before bone marrow transplantation, which includes TBI, induce acute ovarian failure at a very high rate [24, 33].

With respect to premature menopause, radiation to the ovary is associated with the greatest risk of premature menopause [5, 27, 31]. In addition, TBI has also been identified as a severe risk factor for developing premature menopause. In patients older than 10 years, TBI caused premature ovarian failure in over 90% of the patients; in patients younger than 10 years, the ovaries appear more resistant to damage although premature menopause is also frequent in this group [12].

Effect of Chemotherapy

Chemotherapy plays an important role in the treatment of patients with childhood cancer. Alkylating agents are commonly used for childhood sarcomas, leukaemia and lymphomas [34].

Although the pathophysiological mechanisms underlying chemotherapy-induced ovarian failure are not fully understood, they are thought to be related to the cytotoxic actions of the drugs. These can be manifested on the ovaries through impairment of follicular maturation and/or depletion of primordial follicles.

Alkylating agents are the most common chemotherapeutic agents associated with gonadal damage. These agents are not cell cycle-specific and thus do not require cell proliferation for their cytotoxic action. It is believed that they act on undeveloped oocytes and possibly on the pre-granulosa cells of the primordial follicles [30]. By cross-linking DNA and introducing single-strand DNA breaks, alkylating agents destroy cells in a dose-dependent fashion [34]. Cell cycle-specific agents, like anti-metabolites, cause much less gonadotoxicity as their major effect is only on growing and dividing cells affecting ovarian follicle growth and maturation [35].

Treatment with alkylating agents has been associated in many studies among childhood cancer survivors with statistically significant risks for ovarian failure. Both acute effects [25] and effects on (premature) menopause [10, 27, 31] have been described. The highest risks were found in girls treated with the highest cumulative doses of alkylating agents. Studying gonadotoxic effects of individual drugs can be difficult, because many patients receive combination regimens in which several drugs are administered concomitantly. Chemaitilly et al. [25] found a clearly increased risk for treatment with procarbazine and cyclophosphamide. Procarbazine and cyclophosphamide were also found to be associated with significantly increased risks of premature menopause in the cohort of female Hodgkin's survivors described by De Bruin et al. [28]. The risk of procarbazine was dose-dependent [28]. The high risks associated with treatment with busulphan, CCNU and chlorambucil in the study by Chemaitilly et al. [25] were based on very small numbers of exposed patients. Busulphan, however, has also been associated with ovarian failure in several studies including girls that underwent stem cell transplantation [36–38]. Mechlorethamine (nitrogen mustard) is often combined with procarbazine in chemotherapy combination regimens, but seems not to be associated with an independent risk of ovarian failure itself [25, 28].

As previously discussed, acute gonadotoxicity of treatment can differ according to age. Chemaitilly et al. [25] found that treatment with procarbazine is associated with acute ovarian failure regardless of age, whereas treatment with cyclophosphamide only resulted in acute ovarian failure in post-pubertal girls. This is in line with the findings of Sanders et al. [37], who described virtually normal pubertal development among girls treated only with cyclophosphamide in preparation for stem cell transplantation. The fact that the effect of procarbazine is seen in pre-pubertal girls, whereas the effect of cyclophosphamide is not, suggests that procarbazine is more gonadotoxic (in the doses used to treat childhood cancers) than cyclophosphamide. This is in line with the findings from De Bruin et al. [28].

No evidence regarding harmful gonadotoxic effects of non-alkylating chemotherapeutic agents was identified in large studies of childhood cancer survivors with regard to acute ovarian failure [25] and premature menopause [10, 27, 31].

Girls treated with non-alkylating chemotherapy, however, were found to have significantly smaller ovaries and fewer antral follicles compared with controls [5].

Studies that include post-pubertal girls, adolescent and young adult female cancer survivors, and therefore represent a population with a lower baseline ovarian reserve, identified several women experiencing ovarian failure after exposure to non-alkylating agents. However, no significantly increased risks associated with these drugs were identified [28, 29, 39]. The gonadotoxic potential of non-alkylating chemotherapy is therefore regarded to be minimal in girls treated for childhood cancer.

Fertility-Related Late Effects

Treatment for childhood cancer can cause decreased fertility. The decrease itself, however, can cause health-related adverse effects in survivors.

Pregnancy Outcomes

Many studies on pregnancy outcomes of female childhood cancer survivors have been published and reviewed by Green [40]. Two studies on this subject have been performed within the Childhood Cancer Survivor Study [41, 42]. They were large enough to study pregnancy outcomes in relation to treatment. Green et al. [41] studied 4,029 pregnancies in 1,915 female childhood cancer survivors, and found a significantly decreased chance of live birth and an increased risk for miscarriage in most age groups and primary diagnosis strata. Although live births were significantly decreased and miscarriages increased in all broadly defined treatment categories, no differences between the categories were observed. Cranial irradiation was found to be associated with significantly increased risks of miscarriage, especially for miscarriage at 12 or more weeks of gestation. Non-significantly increased rates of miscarriage were found for women whose ovaries were in or near the radiation therapy field. The rate of live births was not lower and the rate of stillbirths was not higher for the patients treated with any particular chemotherapeutic agent. There were also no dose response-related risks for live births or miscarriages identified for any chemotherapeutic agent.

A subgroup of 2,201 singleton live births in 1,264 women was studied by Signorello et al. [42] in more depth with regard to the treatment effects on preterm birth, low birth weight and small gestational age. They found that the children of female childhood cancer survivors were twice as likely to be born preterm as the children of their siblings. The children also had a significantly lower birth weight, but this was attributed to their birth at earlier gestational age. Preterm birth, low birth weight and small gestational age were all significantly associated with radiotherapy to the uterus, but not associated with radiotherapy to the ovaries or the pituitary. The effect of radiotherapy to the uterus was not significantly different for mothers irradiated as pre-pubertal girls compared to post-pubertally irradiated women. Cumulative doses of alkylating chemotherapy showed a non-significant dose-response trend towards more preterm birth among women treated with higher doses. No association with low birth weight or small gestational age of the children was observed.

Although concerns have been raised that potentially mutagenic chemotherapy and radiotherapy may cause germ-line mutations and pose an increased risk of genetic abnormalities in the children born to survivors of cancer, no such evidence has been provided by several large studies on this subject [21, 43].

Premature Menopause and Its Consequences

As discussed above, treatment of childhood cancer can cause premature menopause. Because this permanent cessation of menses can occur not only shortly after treatment, but also later in life at any age before 40 years of age, it can be regarded as a late effect of treatment. The cumulative incidence of premature menopause, occurring 5 years following diagnosis is estimated to be 15% at age 40 [31]. Together with about 6% of women experiencing acute ovarian failure within the first 5 years [25], a substantial proportion of female childhood cancer survivors develop premature menopause. Post-menopausal symptoms include hot flushes, psychosomatic complaints, and sexual dysfunction [44, 45]. Long-term absence of oestrogens can result in increased cholesterol levels, and premature menopause is associated with an increased risk of ischaemic heart disease [45, 46]. In addition, oestrogen is essential in preserving bone mineral density, and premature menopause is associated with osteoporosis [44, 45].

As all these symptoms may have a negative impact on the quality of life and physical well-being of childhood cancer survivors, HRT is often applied in post-menopausal survivors [44, 45]. The use of HRT is regarded as safe in most cancer survivors. With the exception of meningioma, breast and endometrial cancer, there is no biological evidence that HRT may increase recurrence risk [47]. HRT can decrease the risk of osteoporosis [44, 45]. In addition, HRT is found to reduce the increased risk of ischaemic heart disease in women with early menopause [46]. This result is likely to be applicable to female childhood cancer survivors with therapy-induced premature menopause.

The use of HRT, however, is associated with an increased risk of developing hormone-related tumours [47]. Female childhood cancer survivors treated with irradiation to the breast at a young age experience an increased risk for subsequent breast cancer later in life [48]. These are mainly women successfully treated for Hodgkin's lymphoma. Gonadotoxic therapy is found to be associated with a decrease in this increased risk of second breast cancer in adolescent and young adult Hodgkin's survivors [49], but not in childhood cancer survivors [48]. In a subgroup of 185 five-year Hodgkin's survivors treated before age 21 from the Dutch Hodgkin's late effects cohort [28], however, we found that gonadotoxic therapy does lower the risk of breast cancer in these women irradiated to the breast area, but only when menopause is induced relatively shortly after treatment [unpublished data]. In particular, women with <10 years of intact ovarian function after irradiation to the breast, experienced a >10-fold significantly lower risk of subsequent breast cancer compared to those with >20 years of intact ovarian function (HR 0.09, 95% CI 0.01–0.8]. Theoretically it is possible that the beneficial effects of premature menopause on future breast cancer risk in women who received chest irradiation at a young age may be masked by HRT treatment.

Although long-term HRT has a beneficial effect on women's bones, and this beneficial effect is often offset by an increased risk of venous thrombo-embolic disease, breast cancer, stroke, cognitive dysfunction and coronary artery disease [45], the risk-benefit balance for HRT treatment in female childhood cancer survivors has not yet been fully evaluated.

Psychosocial Effects of Fertility Issues

Research on female fertility following cancer treatment during childhood mainly involves the physical effects of cancer and its treatment on reproductive function and ovarian reserve. Little is known about the psychosocial consequences of sub- or infertility or the impact of a history of cancer on the decision of childhood cancer survivors to have children of their own. Available literature suggests nevertheless that having children is important for young cancer survivors [50]. However, many female childhood cancer survivors have little or no knowledge about their fertility status. Zebrack et al. [51] found that 64% of female childhood cancer survivors had no knowledge whatsoever about their fertility status and those who did knew because of a previous or ongoing pregnancy. In addition, many young cancer survivors do not recall ever having talked about the possible impact their former treatment may have on their reproductive capacity [50, 51]. Some do possess or recall information about infertility risks but this information may be inaccurate or dated.

Due to this lack of knowledge, infertility, but also pregnancies, often come as a surprise to many young female cancer survivors. In case of infertility, this inevitably causes significant emotional distress over the loss of a dream to have a child [52]. It is, however, unknown whether the psychological stress of infertility is greater in childhood cancer survivors compared to infertile couples without the history of cancer. One can hypothesise that the burden of infertility may add to the burden of having had cancer causing greater distress in infertile childhood cancer survivors compared to other infertile couples. On the other hand worries about infertility could be more relative in view of the fact that one has survived cancer. There are no studies that have addressed these issues. It has been documented, however, that childhood cancer survivors do worry about their reproductive capacity and/or the health of their offspring, and that females worry more than males [51–53]. The high response rate (85%) to a pilot study in the VU University Medical Centre Amsterdam on reproductive function and ovarian reserve illustrates the need for information regarding this issue amongst female childhood cancer survivors. In addition, Langeveld et al. [53] found that 43% of childhood cancer survivors expressed concerns about the health of their future children, and a similar percentage was reported by Zebrack et al. [51]. This is despite the fact that evidence suggests that children of childhood cancer survivors are not at higher risk of congenital anomalies compared to children of parents without a history of cancer [21, 43]. Appropriate scientific information does not yet sufficiently reach childhood cancer survivors via healthcare professionals although this counselling could possibly reduce fertility-related anxieties.

In addition to worries about the health of their offspring, some childhood cancer survivors have concerns about their own health or their ability to be a good parent [50, 52]. The majority of younger cancer survivors, however, see their cancer experience as potentially making them better parents despite these concerns [50, 51]. Schover et al. [50] reported that 80% of young cancer survivors felt they were or would be good parents in the future. Family life and spending time with family appeared to be very important for cancer survivors and these feelings were specifically attributed to having had cancer [51].

The impact of having had cancer on the decision of childhood cancer survivors to have children of their own seems to be relatively small. Sixteen percent of younger cancer survivors felt a decreased wish to have children due to the impact of cancer. Seventy-one percent did not change their wish and 13% felt an increased wish for children [50]. Only a small percentage of childhood cancer survivors decided to forego having children, but this is not always related to their history of cancer [51].

Even if reproductive function seems to be unaffected by previous cancer treatment and the female survivor, despite her anxieties, does wish to have children, it is important that she is able to engage in an intimate relationship. Studies have suggested that peer relationships, close friendships, self-concept and social competence in non-CNS cancer survivors is relatively similar 2 years after treatment [54]. However, several long-term studies in childhood cancer survivors have shown that the history of cancer has a negative impact on intimate relationships and marriage rates [53–55]. Sharing one's history of cancer with a new partner is particularly relevant for the young adult survivor population and a possible perceived loss of the opportunity to be a parent may be devastating to self-esteem and potentially damaging to marital or other relationships [51]. It has also been reported that childhood cancer survivors are less likely to be sexually active and that they appear to be less satisfied with their interpersonal relationships and sex life [54]. Van Dijk et al. [56] have shown that psychosexual problems are frequent in survivors of childhood cancer. Twenty percent of childhood cancer survivors felt limitations in their sexual life related to the former cancer and the achievement of several psychosexual milestones was delayed [56].

It can be concluded that as the number of female childhood cancer survivors increases, knowledge of the reproductive health status after treatment is becoming more important. Fertility-related concerns are a major source of distress in many young female cancer survivors. Adequate counselling by healthcare professionals is required as is the sharing of available knowledge in order to reduce these fertility-related anxieties.

Options for Fertility Preservation

As described in the previous paragraphs cancer and its treatment may adversely affect fertility and fertility-related issues have been shown to be a source of psychosocial distress in childhood cancer survivors [50, 52]. Information regarding possible treatment-related infertility and available methods to preserve reproductive function is, therefore, essential. However, evidence suggests that the possibility of treatment-related infertility is often not adequately addressed with the patient and/or their parents (in case of a minor) by many (paediatric) oncologists. This may partly be due to lack of knowledge. A study by Goodwin et al. [57] reported that although 90.7% of healthcare providers were aware of the adverse effects of some treatment regimes on fertility, only half were aware of gender differences in gonadotoxicity. In addition, only 53.3% had knowledge of current research and technologies in fertility preservation.

The number of established methods to preserve fertility in female cancer patients is limited, especially in pre-pubertal girls. Several options are available for females but none are as reliable or easy as sperm banking in males and most are still used in an experimental context only. The options available for females are mostly invasive and/or require drug administration. Methods to preserve fertility in females include freezing (embryo cryopreservation, oocyte cryopreservation, ovarian tissue cryopreservation), surgery (ovarian transposition) and/or drug administration (ovarian suppression). Each method has advantages and disadvantages and whether or not an option is suitable for a patient depends on age, diagnosis, type of treatment, time available, the potential that cancer has spread to the ovaries, and the presence of a partner [58]. The different methods of fertility preservation will be briefly described below.

Embryo Cryopreservation

The only currently established method for fertility preservation in females with cancer is the cryopreservation of embryos, a technique routinely used in IVF centres [59]. The human embryo is very resistant to damage caused by cryopreservation. Embryo survival rates after thawing range from 35 to 90% while cumulative pregnancy rates of more than 60% have been described [60, 61].

Despite the fact that this technique has good success rates and is already used in young cancer patients, it also has several disadvantages. The procedure requires ovarian stimulation, oocyte retrieval and IVF. This process takes time (2–6 weeks), which may cause an unacceptable delay in the onset of treatment. In addition, ovarian stimulation is contraindicated in patients with an oestrogen-sensitive tumour, such as breast cancer. Another pitfall of this method is that a partner is required or the female involved must be willing to use donor sperm for fertilisation. Finally, embryo cryopreservation is not an option for pre-pubertal girls with cancer [60, 62].

Cryopreservation of Oocytes

As opposed to embryo cryopreservation, cryopreservation of oocytes (mature and immature) does not require a partner and there may be fewer ethical issues involved [59, 62]. However, compared to embryos, oocytes are much more vulnerable to the freeze-thaw process and the rate of success also depends on the total number of retrieved oocytes [63, 64]. Since the first successful pregnancy in 1986 [65], more than 100 babies have developed from frozen-thawed mature oocytes. However, compared to embryo cryopreservation, pregnancy rates are dramatically low. Sonmezer and Oktay [64] studied data from 21 clinical studies and reported a mean pregnancy rate per thawed oocyte of 1.52%. Even the latest studies show that the overall effectiveness of this technique is very low (<2%/thawed oocyte), despite the fact that the introduction of intra-cytoplasmic sperm injection and recent improvements in the freezing-thawing technique have resulted in somewhat higher survival rates per frozen-thawed oocyte [62, 63, 66].

An additional disadvantage of this technique is that it, like embryo cryopreservation, requires hormonal stimulation of the ovaries which is contraindicated in some types of cancer or can cause a delay in the start of treatment. And finally, this method cannot be used in pre-pubertal girls.

For cryopreservation of oocytes to become a routine clinical procedure research should primarily focus on improving the success rate of the freeze-thaw process in addition to the evaluation of long-term health effects on the offspring born to date from frozen-thawed oocytes.

Cryopreservation of Ovarian Tissue

Until 1999, cryopreservation and autotransplantation of ovarian tissue was performed in animals only. Currently, the technique is still experimental but has led to at least 5 live births in humans [67, 68]. Although there are difficulties, this technique is potentially promising. It is the only option available for females with cancer in whom treatment cannot be delayed. It requires neither ovarian stimulation for the collection of oocytes nor a partner or sperm donor to its success.

Ovarian tissue (either cortical strips or an entire ovary) is collected laparoscopically under general anaesthesia and retrieved fragments of the ovarian cortex are subsequently frozen under strict conditions [62, 63]. Cortical strips contain vast amounts of primordial follicles and their number depends on the age of the patient [33]. Primordial follicles are much more resistant to the freeze-thawing process than mature oocytes and thus survival rates are high [33, 62]. Thawed tissue may subsequently be implanted in the patient, either orthotopically or heterotopically. Many follicles are lost due to the initial tissue ischaemia following transplantation and the survival rate after transplantation is estimated to be approximately 70% [69]. For women over 40 years of age, the benefit of this technique may therefore be limited, since the follicle yield may be too low for it to ever become a success [58]. Despite this follicle loss, recovery of the endocrine and gametogenic function of the ovary has been reported after both orthotopic and heterotopic autotransplantation of ovarian tissue, but live births have been established after orthotopic transplantation only [58, 62, 66–68].

A number of disadvantages with this technique are also recognised. Firstly, the risk of cancer cell reintroduction into the patient must not be ignored, although this risk seems to be relatively small and primarily restricted to blood-borne cancers such as leukaemia and lymphoma [66, 70]. Secondly, both laparoscopy and the general anaesthesia under which this intervention is performed have recognised morbidity rates. And finally, one must be vigilant for the transmission of viral diseases and the contamination of storage facilities [33].

Apart from women in whom treatment cannot be delayed, this method is also the only method available for pre-pubertal girls. In a recent study of 49 prepubertal girls due to receive potentially sterilising cancer therapy, Poirot et al. [71]

reported ovarian tissue cryopreservation to be highly feasible, safe, and acceptable to most patients and/or their families. In addition, it did not delay treatment. They concluded that cryopreservation of ovarian tissue could be systematically offered even to pre-pubertal girls at risk of sterility due to cancer treatment. These findings are in line with guidelines suggested by Weintraub et al. [72].

In conclusion, although ovarian tissue cryopreservation appears to be a safe, easy and relatively inexpensive procedure to potentially preserve female fertility, even in pre-pubertal girls, the efficacy and reliability of this method as well as the crucial issues of tissue ischaemia and cancer cell reintroduction need to be addressed in future research.

Ovarian Suppression with GnRH Analogues or Antagonists

Suppressing ovarian function by inhibition of the pituitary through the use of GnRH analogues in order to ultimately preserve fertility is a controversial method of fertility preservation, and studies in humans are limited. Some small studies render a positive effect while others show no benefit [58, 66]. In a recent study Blumenfeld et al. [70] assessed the gonadotoxic effect of chemotherapy with or without concomitant treatment with a GnRH agonist. It is the largest prospective study to date evaluating long-term ovarian function (follow-up between 2 and 15 years) in 111 female Hodgkin's lymphoma patients. Sixty-five patients received GnRH agonist treatment next to their CT treatment, 96.9% of whom resumed ovulation and regular menses compared to 3% of the controls. The number of spontaneous pregnancies were, however, not significantly different between the 2 groups.

These data suggest that ovarian damage in female patients treated for Hodgkin's lymphoma may be significantly reduced by co-treatment with GnRH agonists [70]. Therefore, GnRH co-treatment should be considered in addition to other methods of fertility preservation in women receiving gonadotoxic treatment. Combining the various modalities for a specific patient may increase the odds for preservation of future fertility [70]. GnRH analogues do not, however, protect primordial follicles from radiation damage [62].

The protective role of GnRH antagonists has been studied in animals only and data are not very promising [70].

Ovarian Transposition (Oophoropexy)

Radiotherapy may have devastating effects on the primordial follicle pool in the ovaries resulting in infertility and premature ovarian failure. An established method to physically preserve fertility from radiotherapy to the pelvic area is oophoropexy: moving the ovaries as far out of the radiation field as possible.

Nowadays, transpositioning of the ovaries is mainly performed by laparoscopy. It is a safe, simple and effective technique which causes no delay in treatment and less adhesions compared to the previously used technique (laparotomy) [62]. The dose of radiotherapy to the ovary is reduced to 5–10% of the dose the ovary would have received in situ. Rates of ovarian preservation and the ability to conceive vary between 16–90% [66] and depend on the degree of scatter radiation, the presence of vascular compromise, the age of the patient, the dose of radiation, whether the ovaries are shielded, and whether concomitant chemotherapy is given [61].

The technique also has several disadvantages. Firstly, the procedure is not always reliable since the ovaries may migrate back to its original position and complications may occur [62]. Secondly, the method is only of value to patients receiving radiotherapy to the pelvic area. It does not protect the ovaries against the gonadotoxic effects of chemotherapy. Finally, even if the procedure is successful in preserving ovarian function, fertility may be compromised if the uterus remains in the radiation field.

In conclusion, although embryo cryopreservation is still the only established method for fertility preservation in female cancer patients, other experimental techniques show promising results. The prospects for ovarian tissue cryopreservation with subsequent autotransplantation are exciting and the technique has been shown not only to be feasible and safe in adult females of reproductive age but also in pre-pubertal girls. In addition, combining options of fertility preservation in order to increase a woman's chance of becoming a mother should not be overlooked.

References

1 Tilly JL, Johnson J: Recent arguments against germ cell renewal in the adult human ovary: is an absence of marker gene expression really acceptable evidence of an absence of oogenesis? Cell Cycle 2007;6:879–883.

2 Faddy MJ, Gosden RG: A mathematical model of follicle dynamics in the human ovary. Hum Reprod 1995;10:770–775.

3 Lutchman SK, Davies M, Chatterjee R: Fertility in female cancer survivors: pathophysiology, preservation and the role of ovarian reserve testing. Hum Reprod Update 2005;11:69–89.

4 Wallace WH, Anderson RA, Irvine DS: Fertility preservation for young patients with cancer: who is at risk and what can be offered? Lancet Oncol 2005;6:209–218.

5 Larsen EC, Muller J, Schmiegelow K, Rechnitzer C, Andersen AN: Reduced ovarian function in long-term survivors of radiation- and chemotherapy-treated childhood cancer. J Clin Endocrinol Metab 2003;88:5307–5314.

6 Howell S, Shalet S: Gonadal damage from chemotherapy and radiotherapy. Endocrinol Metab Clin North Am 1998;27:927–943.

7 Broekmans FJ, Kwee J, Hendriks DJ, Mol BW, Lambalk CB: A systematic review of tests predicting ovarian reserve and IVF outcome. Hum Reprod Update 2006;12:685–718.

8 National Collaborating Centre for Women's and Children's Health: Fertility: Assessment and Treatment for People with Fertility Problems. Clinical Guideline 11. London, National Institute for Clinical Excellence, 2004.

9 Critchley HO, Bath LE, Wallace WH: Radiation damage to the uterus – review of the effects of treatment of childhood cancer. Hum Fertil (Camb) 2002;5:61–66.
10 Byrne J, Fears TR, Gail MH, et al: Early menopause in long-term survivors of cancer during adolescence. Am J Obstet Gynecol 1992;166:788–793.
11 Gleeson HK, Shalet SM: The impact of cancer therapy on the endocrine system in survivors of childhood brain tumours. Endocr Relat Cancer 2004;11:589–602.
12 Critchley HO, Wallace WH: Impact of cancer treatment on uterine function. J Natl Cancer Inst Monogr 2005;34:64–68.
13 Chow EJ, Friedman DL, Yasui Y, et al: Timing of menarche among survivors of childhood acute lymphoblastic leukemia: a report from the Childhood Cancer Survivor Study. Pediatr Blood Cancer 2008;50:854–858.
14 Livesey EA, Brook CG: Gonadal dysfunction after treatment of intracranial tumours. Arch Dis Child 1988;63:495–500.
15 Bath LE, Anderson RA, Critchley HO, Kelnar CJ, Wallace WH: Hypothalamic-pituitary-ovarian dysfunction after prepubertal chemotherapy and cranial irradiation for acute leukaemia. Hum Reprod 2001;16:1838–1844.
16 Baird DD, Weinberg CR, Zhou H, et al: Preimplantation urinary hormone profiles and the probability of conception in healthy women. Fertil Steril 1999;71:40–49.
17 Soules MR, McLachlan RI, Ek M, Dahl KD, Cohen NL, Bremner WJ: Luteal phase deficiency: characterization of reproductive hormones over the menstrual cycle. J Clin Endocrinol Metab 1989;69:804–812.
18 Critchley HO, Wallace WH, Shalet SM, Mamtora H, Higginson J, Anderson DC: Abdominal irradiation in childhood; the potential for pregnancy. Br J Obstet Gynaecol 1992;99:392–394.
19 Bath LE, Critchley HO, Chambers SE, Anderson RA, Kelnar CJ, Wallace WH: Ovarian and uterine characteristics after total body irradiation in childhood and adolescence: response to sex steroid replacement. Br J Obstet Gynaecol 1999;106:1265–1272.
20 Holm K, Nysom K, Brocks V, Hertz H, Jacobsen N, Muller J: Ultrasound B-mode changes in the uterus and ovaries and Doppler changes in the uterus after total body irradiation and allogeneic bone marrow transplantation in childhood. Bone Marrow Transplant 1999;23:259–263.
21 Edgar AB, Wallace WH: Pregnancy in women who had cancer in childhood. Eur J Cancer 2007;43:1890–1894.
22 Critchley HO, Buckley CH, Anderson DC: Experience with a 'physiological' steroid replacement regimen for the establishment of a receptive endometrium in women with premature ovarian failure. Br J Obstet Gynaecol 1990;97:804–810.
23 Larsen EC, Schmiegelow K, Rechnitzer C, Loft A, Muller J, Andersen AN: Radiotherapy at a young age reduces uterine volume of childhood cancer survivors. Acta Obstet Gynecol Scand 2004;83:96–102.
24 Sklar C: Maintenance of ovarian function and risk of premature menopause related to cancer treatment. J Natl Cancer Inst Monogr 2005;34:25–27.
25 Chemaitilly W, Mertens AC, Mitby P, et al: Acute ovarian failure in the childhood cancer survivor study. J Clin Endocrinol Metab 2006;91:1723–1728.
26 Sanders JE, Buckner CD, Amos D, et al: Ovarian function following marrow transplantation for aplastic anemia or leukemia. J Clin Oncol 1988;6:813–818.
27 Chiarelli AM, Marrett LD, Darlington G: Early menopause and infertility in females after treatment for childhood cancer diagnosed in 1964–1988 in Ontario, Canada. Am J Epidemiol 1999;150:245–254.
28 De Bruin ML, Huisbrink J, Hauptmann M, et al: Treatment-related risk factors for premature menopause following Hodgkin lymphoma. Blood 2008;111:101–108.
29 Haukvik UK, Dieset I, Bjoro T, Holte H, Fossa SD: Treatment-related premature ovarian failure as a long-term complication after Hodgkin's lymphoma. Ann Oncol 2006;17:1428–1433.
30 Blumenfeld Z, Avivi I, Ritter M, Rowe JM: Preservation of fertility and ovarian function and minimizing chemotherapy-induced gonadotoxicity in young women. J Soc Gynecol Investig 1999;6:229–239.
31 Sklar CA, Mertens AC, Mitby P, et al: Premature menopause in survivors of childhood cancer: a report from the childhood cancer survivor study. J Natl Cancer Inst 2006;98:890–896.
32 Wallace WH, Thomson AB, Kelsey TW: The radiosensitivity of the human oocyte. Hum Reprod 2003;18:117–121.
33 Bath LE, Wallace WH, Critchley HO: Late effects of the treatment of childhood cancer on the female reproductive system and the potential for fertility preservation. BJOG 2002;109:107–114.

34 Gracia CR, Ginsberg JP: Fertility risk in pediatric and adolescent cancers. Cancer Treat Res 2007;138:57–72.
35 Hensley ML, Reichman BS: Fertility and pregnancy after adjuvant chemotherapy for breast cancer. Crit Rev Oncol Hematol 1998;28:121–128.
36 Sanders JE, Hawley J, Levy W, et al: Pregnancies following high-dose cyclophosphamide with or without high-dose busulfan or total-body irradiation and bone marrow transplantation. Blood 1996;87:3045–3052.
37 Sanders ME, Scroggins T, Ampil FL, Li BD: Accelerated partial breast irradiation in early-stage breast cancer. J Clin Oncol 2007;25:996–1002.
38 Thibaud E, Rodriguez-Macias K, Trivin C, Esperou H, Michon J, Brauner R: Ovarian function after bone marrow transplantation during childhood. Bone Marrow Transplant 1998;21:287–290.
39 Meirow D: Reproduction post-chemotherapy in young cancer patients. Mol Cell Endocrinol 2000;169:123–131.
40 Green DM: Pregnancy outcome; in Wallace WH, Green DM (eds): Late Effects of Childhood Cancer. London, Hodder Education, 2003, pp 257–266.
41 Green DM, Whitton JA, Stovall M, et al: Pregnancy outcome of female survivors of childhood cancer: a report from the Childhood Cancer Survivor Study. Am J Obstet Gynecol 2002;187:1070–1080.
42 Signorello LB, Cohen SS, Bosetti C, et al: Female survivors of childhood cancer: preterm birth and low birth weight among their children. J Natl Cancer Inst 2006;98:1453–1461.
43 Byrne J, Rasmussen SA, Steinhorn SC, et al: Genetic disease in offspring of long-term survivors of childhood and adolescent cancer. Am J Hum Genet 1998;62:45–52.
44 Clemons M, Clamp A, Anderson B: Management of the menopause in cancer survivors. Cancer Treat Rev 2002;28:321–333.
45 Molina JR, Barton DL, Loprinzi CL: Chemotherapy-induced ovarian failure: manifestations and management. Drug Saf 2005;28:401–416.
46 Lokkegaard E, Jovanovic Z, Heitmann BL, Keiding N, Ottesen B, Pedersen AT: The association between early menopause and risk of ischaemic heart disease: influence of hormone therapy. Maturitas 2006;53:226–233.
47 Biglia N, Gadducci A, Ponzone R, Roagna R, Sismondi P: Hormone replacement therapy in cancer survivors. Maturitas 2004;48:333–346.
48 Kenney LB, Yasui Y, Inskip PD, et al: Breast cancer after childhood cancer: a report from the Childhood Cancer Survivor Study. Ann Intern Med 2004;141:590–597.
49 van Leeuwen FE, Klokman WJ, Stovall M, et al: Roles of radiation dose, chemotherapy, and hormonal factors in breast cancer following Hodgkin's disease. J Natl Cancer Inst 2003;95:971–980.
50 Schover LR, Rybicki LA, Martin BA, Bringelsen KA. Having children after cancer. A pilot survey of survivors' attitudes and experiences. Cancer 1999;86:697–709.
51 Zebrack BJ, Casillas J, Nohr L, Adams H, Zeltzer LK: Fertility issues for young adult survivors of childhood cancer. Psychooncology 2004;13:689–699.
52 Schover LR: Psychosocial aspects of infertility and decisions about reproduction in young cancer survivors: a review. Med Pediatr Oncol 1999;33:53–59.
53 Langeveld NE, Grootenhuis MA, Voute PA, de Haan RJ, van den BC: Quality of life, self-esteem and worries in young adult survivors of childhood cancer. Psychooncology 2004;13:867–881.
54 Gerhardt CA, Vannatta K, Valerius KS, Correll J, Noll RB: Social and romantic outcomes in emerging adulthood among survivors of childhood cancer. J Adolesc Health 2007;40:462–415.
55 Joubert D, Sadeghi MR, Elliott M, Devins GM, Laperriere N, Rodin G: Physical sequelae and self-perceived attachment in adult survivors of childhood cancer. Psychooncology 2001;10:284–292.
56 van Dijk EM, van Dulmen-den Broeder E, Kaspers GJ, van Dam EW, Braam KI, Huisman J: Psychosexual functioning of childhood cancer survivors. Psychooncology 2008;17:506–511.
57 Goodwin T, Elizabeth OB, Kiernan M, Hudson MM, Dahl GV: Attitudes and practices of pediatric oncology providers regarding fertility issues. Pediatr Blood Cancer 2007;48:80–85.
58 Lee SJ, Schover LR, Partridge AH, et al: American Society of Clinical Oncology recommendations on fertility preservation in cancer patients. J Clin Oncol 2006;24:2917–2931.
59 Ethics Committee of the American Society for Reproductive Medicine: Fertility preservation and reproduction in cancer patients. Fertil Steril 2005;83:1622–1628.
60 Maltaris T, Boehm D, Dittrich R, Seufert R, Koelbl H: Reproduction beyond cancer: a message of hope for young women. Gynecol Oncol 2006;103:1109–1121.

61 Marhhom E, Cohen I: Fertility preservation options for women with malignancies. Obstet Gynecol Surv 2007;62:58–72.

62 Kim SS: Fertility preservation in female cancer patients: current developments and future directions. Fertil Steril 2006;85:1–11.

63 Donnez J, Martinez-Madrid B, Jadoul P, Van LA, Demylle D, Dolmans MM: Ovarian tissue cryopreservation and transplantation: a review. Hum Reprod Update 2006;12:519–535.

64 Sonmezer M, Oktay K: Fertility preservation in female patients. Hum Reprod Update 2004;10: 251–266.

65 Chen C: Pregnancy after human oocyte cryopreservation. Lancet 1986;i:884–886.

66 Maltaris T, Seufert R, Fischl F, et al: The effect of cancer treatment on female fertility and strategies for preserving fertility. Eur J Obstet Gynecol Reprod Biol 2007;130:148–155.

67 Donnez J, Dolmans MM, Demylle D, et al: Livebirth after orthotopic transplantation of cryopreserved ovarian tissue. Lancet 2004;364:1405–1410.

68 Meirow D, Levron J, Eldar-Geva T, et al: Pregnancy after transplantation of cryopreserved ovarian tissue in a patient with ovarian failure after chemotherapy. N Engl J Med 2005;353:318–321.

69 Oktay K, Nugent D, Newton H, Salha O, Chatterjee P, Gosden RG: Isolation and characterization of primordial follicles from fresh and cryopreserved human ovarian tissue. Fertil Steril 1997;67: 481–486.

70 Blumenfeld Z, Avivi I, Eckman A, Epelbaum R, Rowe JM, Dann EJ: Gonadotropin-releasing hormone agonist decreases chemotherapy-induced gonadotoxicity and premature ovarian failure in young female patients with Hodgkin lymphoma. Fertil Steril 2008;89:166–173.

71 Poirot CJ, Martelli H, Genestie C, et al: Feasibility of ovarian tissue cryopreservation for prepubertal females with cancer. Pediatr Blood Cancer 2007; 49:74–78.

72 Weintraub M, Gross E, Kadari A, et al: Should ovarian cryopreservation be offered to girls with cancer. Pediatr Blood Cancer 2007;48:4–9.

Marie L. De Bruin, PhD
Department of Epidemiology, Netherlands Cancer Institute
Plesmanlaan 121
NL–1066 CX Amsterdam (The Netherlands)
Tel. +31 20 512 2480, Fax +31 20 512 2322, E-Mail m.d.bruin@nki.nl

Wallace WHB, Kelnar CJH (eds): Endocrinopathy after Childhood Cancer Treatment.
Endocr Dev. Basel, Karger, 2009, vol 15, pp 159–180

Long-Term Follow-Up of Survivors of Childhood Cancer

Angela B. Edgar[a] · Elizabeth M.M. Morris[b] · Christopher J.H. Kelnar[c] · W. Hamish B. Wallace[a]

[a]Department of Oncology, Royal Hospital for Sick Children, [b]Hermitage Medical Practices and [c]Section of Child Life and Health, Division of Reproductive and Developmental Sciences, University of Edinburgh, Edinburgh, UK

Abstract

Today more than 75% of children treated for cancer will be cured, and attention is focusing on the late effects of treatments for these long-term survivors. Treatment-related morbidity is diverse, with potential effects on the endocrine system (growth, puberty, fertility, pituitary, thyroid and other disorders), cardiovascular, pulmonary and renal complications, second tumours, cognitive, education, neuropsychological and social manifestations. Multi-disciplinary long-term follow-up of these patients is essential to monitor, treat, and prevent morbidity. Depending on the nature of the treatment delivered, long-term follow-up of the survivor of childhood cancer can be individualised and delivered by a wide range of health professionals either in hospital or in primary care. In this review we describe the chronic health problems encountered by survivors and discuss the development of a long-term follow-up service for childhood cancer survivors.

Cancer in childhood is relatively uncommon, with about 1,400 new cases per year in the UK, and a cumulative risk of 1 in 600 by the age of 15 years. Therapeutic advances and specialist cancer centres mean that the majority of children can realistically hope for long-term survival. With survival rates currently in the region of 75%, it has been estimated that by 2010, 1 in 715 of the young adult population will be a long-term survivor of childhood cancer [1]. Cure is generally achieved with multi-agent chemotherapy, plus or minus surgery, radiotherapy and bone marrow or stem cell transplantation, but is frequently associated with late effects and morbidity. The North American Childhood Cancer Survivor Study (CCSS), which has studied long-term health outcomes in more than 20,000 long-term survivors of childhood cancer, has reported a standardised mortality ratio of 10.8 for the whole cohort when compared to age-matched normal controls, of which cancer recurrence accounted for two thirds of the deaths and about 20% were complications related to treatment [2, 3]. Treatment-related morbidity is diverse and may give rise to endocrine dysfunction (including growth impairment, infertility, hypothyroidism), cardiovascular disease, pulmonary and renal complications, cognitive impairment, educational problems, neuropsychological difficulties, and social problems. It has recently been reported in the UK that almost 75% of childhood cancer survivors have one or more chronic health problems, 40% have suffered at least one life-threatening/disabling event, and 25% of survivors have at least five chronic health problems [4].

Today paediatric oncologists are faced with the challenge of sustaining the excellent survival rates whilst striving to achieve optimal quality of life. Late effects may occur soon after treatment or may not present for many years. Life-long follow-up of survivors is recommended and this will necessitate multidisciplinary collaboration between oncologists and other health professionals to ensure early diagnosis, counselling and, where possible, timely institution of appropriate treatments [5–8]. The need to develop guidelines for the assessment of late effects of cancer therapy is reflected in recently published guidelines from the US Children's Oncology Group, the UK National Institute for Clinical Excellence (NICE), the Scottish Intercollegiate Guidelines Network (SIGN) and the UK Children's Cancer and Leukaemia Group (CCLG).

This chapter will describe the chronic health problems encountered by survivors and discuss strategies for the development of a long-term follow-up service. In particular, we focus on an evidence-based approach developed by SIGN and discuss how this is complemented by other guidelines [9]. The SIGN guideline provides a systematic review of the evidence available in five areas of long-term follow-up [9, 10]. These are: (1) the assessment and achievement of normal growth; (2) achievement of normal progression through puberty and factors affecting fertility; (3) early identification, assessment and treatment of cardiac abnormalities; (4) assessment of thyroid function, and (5) assessment and achievement of optimum neurodevelopment and psychological health. (Based upon the evidence available, SIGN guidance provides a grade of recommendation to guide the management decisions: reflecting the strength of the evidence on which the recommendation is based and does not reflect the clinical importance of the recommendation.) Other important areas not addressed by the guideline include renal, respiratory and liver dysfunction, second malignancies, and visual and hearing impairment. It is planned that a future SIGN guideline will address these issues. Each of the five areas covered in the guideline, with brief mention of the other areas, is discussed below.

Endocrine Function

Disorders of the endocrine system are commonly encountered in up to 50% of childhood cancer survivors following chemotherapy and radiotherapy, and include growth impairment, thyroid dysfunction, disrupted puberty and infertility [11].

Hypothalamic-Pituitary Dysfunction

Children who receive cranial irradiation for brain tumours, nasopharyngeal carcinoma, acute lymphoblastic leukaemia (ALL) or total body irradiation in preparation for bone marrow transplant are at risk of developing hypothalamic-pituitary dysfunction (hypopituitarism) and multiple pituitary hormone deficiencies [11–18]. The extent and timing of onset of these disorders is related to the total dose of irradiation, fractionation schedule and time from treatment. The hypothalamus is more radiosensitive than the pituitary [18, but also see Darzy and Shalet, pp 1–24]. The frequency and severity of hypothalamic-pituitary dysfunction increase with time after irradiation due to secondary pituitary atrophy [15]. Growth hormone (GH) is the most vulnerable anterior pituitary hormone to irradiation, followed by gonadotrophin, corticotrophins and thyrotrophin [15, 16]. Isolated GH deficiency may develop 10 or more years after fractionated doses as low as 10–12 Gy while higher doses (over 60 Gy) may produce panhypopituitarism [17, 18]. Patients treated for ALL with prophylactic cranial irradiation (18–24 Gy) have been found to have abnormalities of GH secretion up to 25 years following treatment. Treatment of nasopharyngeal tumours or brain tumours exposes patients to much higher doses of irradiation and is associated with GH deficiency in 50% of patients within 5 years, and is often compounded by other pituitary deficiencies [19].

Growth Problems

Treatment with chemotherapy and radiotherapy may have a significant impact on the growth and development of the child and short stature is well documented following cranial and craniospinal irradiation. Growth may be impaired as a result of GH insufficiency (compounded by other pituitary hormone deficiencies), impaired spinal growth, disrupted bone mineral homeostasis, immobilisation, and nutritional problems [11–18].

Radiotherapy to the spine (for CNS tumour or abdominal irradiation) may have a direct impact on spinal growth by causing permanent disruption to the epiphyses. The damage is greater with single dose versus fractionated irradiation and with younger age at the time of treatment [16, 17]. The spinal growth spurt occurs towards the end of secondary sexual development, therefore, radiotherapy to the spine will result in late pubertal growth failure.

Younger children, especially girls, are more likely to develop early or precocious puberty and a pubertal growth spurt can be mistaken for 'catch-up' growth [10]. Obesity can normalise growth at the expense of a disproportionate bone age advance and reduce final height.

Bone development is maximal during puberty and peak bone mass is reached in the third decade of life. Evaluation of bone mineral density in long-term survivors of ALL has shown reduced bone mineral density [20, 21]. Although this is likely to be multifactorial, involving a combination of alterations in calcium absorption, vitamin D metabolism, IGF-binding proteins and GH insufficiency, there is increasing evidence to implicate chemotherapy. At presentation with ALL there is already low bone turnover with reduced levels of collagen formation and resorption markers (PICP, PIIINP and ICTP) [21]. In remission, there is further suppression of bone synthesis (low levels of PICP and PIIINP) and growth suppression that probably relates to glucocorticoid (prednisolone) and high dose methotrexate therapies [22–25]. Reduced bone mineral density will increase the risk of osteopenia, osteoporosis and pathological fractures in later life.

Management of Growth

It is recommended that all children should undergo regular assessment of growth (sitting and standing height, skin folds, weight, BMI and pubertal staging) until final height is reached (SIGN grade B recommendation). Children with craniopharyngioma or impaired growth should undergo assessment of pituitary function with appropriate stimulation tests. Children with impaired growth velocity should have GH levels measured after appropriate stimulation tests (SIGN grade C recommendation). Children with a good prognosis 2 years out from treatment with proven GH deficiency should have GH replacement therapy (SIGN grade B recommendation). The relapse rate is higher in the first 2 years after diagnosis, and there is no evidence that GH is associated with reactivation of the primary lesion [26]. Children with craniopharyngioma may need GH from presentation (SIGN grade B recommendation) and GH response is similar to that seen in children with idiopathic GH deficiency. Where the cause of growth impairment is unclear, a trial of GH may be appropriate (SIGN grade C recommendation). Young girls receiving cranial radiotherapy should be monitored for precocious puberty (SIGN grade B recommendation).

Obesity

Survivors (especially girls and those with ALL, brain tumours and craniopharyngioma) are at risk of obesity in adolescence and adult life. The aetiology is multifactorial (nutritional, psychological, lifestyle including lack of exercise, endocrine and neuroendocrine) and is difficult to identify or treat [27, 28]. The consequences of childhood obesity are multiple, with an adverse impact on educational attainment and interpersonal relationships, especially in males. Monitoring of weight and calculation of BMI should be carried out routinely. Advice on healthy eating and exercise should be given early and reinforced regularly [Gregory, pp 59–76].

Thyroid Disorders

Thyroid disorders are commonly encountered following radiation treatment for cancer, either secondary to disruption of the hypothalamic-pituitary-thyroid axis or following direct damage to the thyroid gland itself. Thyroid gland abnormalities may present as thyroid dysfunction, nodules and, rarely, thyroid cancer [29, 30]. Central hypothyroidism with TSH deficiency, may develop following cranial or craniospinal irradiation, although it is uncommon with doses of <40 Gy. However, there is some evidence to suggest that lower doses may be associated with clinically significant subtle damage to thyrotrophin secretion despite apparently normal biochemical levels of TSH and thyroid hormone. Direct damage to the thyroid gland following radiation of the neck, at a fractionated dose of >18 Gy, most commonly presents as hypothyroidism, with low T_4 and elevated TSH. Risk factors are radiation dose, female sex, and older age at diagnosis, with the highest risk 5 years after irradiation [31]. Chemotherapy is an independent risk factor for thyroid dysfunction and may potentiate radiation-induced damage. Hyperthyroidism may also develop from about 8 years after irradiation at doses of >35 Gy, but this is less common [30].

Irradiation involving the neck also confers an increased risk of developing both benign and malignant thyroid tumours. The risk of developing thyroid tumours increases with radiation dose, younger age at the time of treatment and female gender [32]. In the past, children treated with low dose radiotherapy for a variety of non-thyroid malignant disorders, including lymphoid hyperplasia and various skin conditions, have a significantly increased risk of thyroid cancer (<10% over 35 years) [33]. Radiation-induced thyroid cancers were all too evident following the devastating impact of the radioactive fallout from the Chernobyl nuclear power plant accident in 1986. Thyroid nodules may be benign (adenomas, focal hyperplasia and colloid nodules), or malignant, most frequently papillary carcinoma secondary to irradiation, which is highly curable if detected early.

It is recommended that survivors of childhood cancer who have received radiotherapy to the neck, brain or spine should have thyroid function checked at the end of treatment and at regular intervals thereafter for life (SIGN grade B recommendations). There are no good quality studies that address the question of screening for thyroid nodules or second primary thyroid cancers. At-risk survivors should be advised accordingly and asked to seek urgent medical advice if they notice a palpable neck mass.

Thyroid hormone replacement therapy is safe and effective, although cautious introduction is necessary in patients treated with anthracyclines who are at risk of cardiac dysfunction. There is no evidence to support or refute the use of thyroxine in compensated hypothyroidism, although it is arguable that supplementation is warranted in these patients as hyperstimulation with persistently elevated TSH may theoretically predispose to malignant change.

Hypothalamic-Pituitary-Adrenal Axis

The hypothalamic-pituitary-adrenal axis has been shown to be relatively radioresistant. ACTH deficiency is potentially a life-threatening condition, often with subtle onset, which although rare following low-dose cranial irradiation must be considered in patients with pituitary tumours or those receiving cranial irradiation doses in excess of 50 Gy [15]. The insulin tolerance test is regarded as the gold standard for assessing the integrity of the hypothalamic-pituitary-adrenal axis, although severe hypoglycaemia may be problematic. Subtle clinical signs and diagnostic difficulties may lead to an underestimation of the true incidence of abnormalities of the hypothalamic-pituitary-adrenal axis. However, once identified, life-long hydrocortisone replacement is required and increased doses may be necessary for surgery or inter-current illness.

Hypothalamic-Pituitary-Gonadal Axis

The impact of cranial irradiation on the hypothalamic-pituitary gonadal axis is complex [Darzy and Shalet, pp 1–24; Armstrong et al., pp 25–39], and the clinical manifestations are dependent upon the dose received and gender of the patient. Relatively high doses of cranial irradiation may disrupt the hypothalamic-pituitary-gonadal axis resulting in hypogonadism. The hypothalamus is more radiosensitive than the pituitary gland with hypothalamic GnRH deficiency being the most frequent aetiology. Radiation doses of 35–45 Gy are associated with impaired gonadotropin secretion with increasing time following radiation [15, 34]. Clinical manifestations vary from subclinical biochemical abnormalities, detectable only on GnRH stimulation to clinically obvious delayed puberty and impaired reproductive function, readily treated with hormone replacement therapy. However, precocious puberty may also occur in both boys and especially girls following high doses or cranial irradiation for brain tumours, and is more profound the younger the patients at the time of treatment [35]. To further complicate matters this early onset of puberty may be followed by the evolution of gonadotropin deficiency, necessitating the judicious use of gonadotropin analogues to suppress pubertal development. Early pubertal development is also associated with a premature growth spurt and early epiphyseal fusion and reduced final adult height.

In contrast, low dose cranial irradiation (18–24 Gy; 2-Gy fractions), as part of CNS-directed therapy in children with ALL prior to 1992, was associated with precocious puberty, predominantly affecting girls [36]. This highlights the differential effects of radiotherapy and the sex differences in the regulation of pubertal development. However, following low dose cranial radiotherapy (18–24 Gy), a subtle decline in hypothalamic-pituitary ovarian function may occur with time, posing a clinical challenge. Decreased LH secretion, an attenuated LH surge, and shorter luteal phases have been reported and may herald incipient ovarian failure or be associated with early pregnancy loss [37].

High dose radiotherapy (>24 Gy) for brain tumours may disrupt hypothalamic/pituitary function and result in delayed puberty, whereas lower doses (<24 Gy) are more commonly associated with precocious puberty, especially if treated when very young [35]. This is most commonly seen in children who received cranial irradiation as CNS-directed treatment for ALL. The subsequent pubertal growth spurt can be mistaken for 'catch-up' growth.

Reproductive Function and Health of the Offspring

One of the most frequently encountered and psychologically traumatic late complications following treatment for childhood cancer is infertility. Cytotoxic therapy may damage gonadal tissue at all ages and result in permanent sterility in both males and females. A number of chemotherapy agents are known to be gonadotoxic and modern treatment regimens are being introduced to minimise the risk of infertility. Previous treatment of Hodgkin's lymphoma in the UK with ChlVPP (chlorambucil, vinblastine, procarbazine, prednisolone) was associated with almost universal permanent sterility in males and raised gonadotrophins in around 50% of females, which with time may manifest as a premature menopause [38]. Current UK treatment with OEPA (vincristine, etoposide, prednisolone and doxorubicin) +/− radiotherapy is likely to be less gonadotoxic.

The extent of radiation damage to the reproductive tissue depends on the radiation dose, fractionation schedule and age at the time of treatment. In males, the testicular germinal epithelium is more susceptible than the testosterone-producing Leydig cells. Permanent azoospermia may follow a single fraction of 4 Gy, while testosterone insufficiency ensues after doses of >20 Gy in pre-pubertal boys and >30 Gy in post-pubertal men [39–43]. Therefore, secondary sexual development and potency may be preserved despite infertility. Spontaneously conceived offspring of cancer survivors have no excess of congenital anomalies or other diseases [44, 45]. Advances in assisted reproductive techniques, particularly intracytoplasmic sperm injection, make paternity achievable for men with low sperm counts. Although the best available data on the health of offspring following intracytoplasmic sperm injection are broadly reassuring [46], there are no data on the health of the offspring where the man's deficit in semen quality is a consequence of potentially mutagenic treatment. Reassuringly, despite cancer therapy-induced oligozoospermia, the healthy sperm DNA is comparable to the normal population.

In females, the primordial follicle is very sensitive to radiation, with an estimated LD_{50} of <2 Gy [48]. The number of primordial follicles present at the time of treatment is age-dependent, and the total dose received will determine the fertile 'window' and influence the age of premature ovarian failure [49]. Uterine radiation in childhood increases the incidence of nulliparity, spontaneous miscarriage and intrauterine growth retardation, probably attributable to reduced uterine musculature elasticity and vascular damage [50–53].

As with males there is the theoretical risk that exposure to chemotherapeutic agents and irradiation may cause mutations and DNA changes to the oocyte. Animal studies have demonstrated high abortion and malformation rates related to different stages of oocyte maturation at the time of exposure to chemotherapy. This has raised concerns regarding the use of assisted reproduction techniques and embryo cryopreservation in patients previously exposed to cancer therapy. Reassuringly, studies of pregnancy outcome in cancer survivors have not substantiated these concerns [44, 45, 53]. There is no increased incidence of chromosomal or congenital abnormalities in the offspring born to women exposed to cancer therapy. Children born following assisted conception using spermatozoa and immature spermatogenic cells require careful long-term monitoring.

Monitoring Pubertal Development and Assessing Reproductive Function

All children should have assessment of gonadal function as part of routine follow-up. In males it is recommended that clinical examination includes Tanner staging of secondary sexual characteristics and assessment of testicular volume using the Prader orchidometer. A testicular volume of <12 ml strongly correlates with impaired spermatogenesis. Hormone assessments of serum FSH/LH/testosterone should also be routinely performed. Inhibin B seems to be a sensitive guide to Sertoli cell damage in adult men but not in prepubertal boys [54]. Semen analysis is the gold standard for Sertoli cell function and should be offered and encouraged at the appropriate time. Fertility counselling should be provided for survivors of childhood cancer. Men demonstrating evidence of impaired fertility should be referred to a clinical andrologist for further assessment as they may benefit from assisted reproductive technology.

Girls treated with cranial irradiation should have their pubertal status assessed three to four times per year from the end of treatment as part of routine clinical assessment (SIGN grade C recommendation). Early follicular phase assay of FSH, oestradiol and inhibin B and ovarian ultrasound are potential tools to assess ovarian reserve. Women who have evidence of impaired fertility should be referred for specialist assessment as they could benefit from assisted reproductive technology (SIGN grade C recommendation).

Preservation of fertility is dictated by sexual maturity with the only available established options being cryopreservation of spermatozoa in the male and embryos for the female with a partner, with the latter clearly not an option for paediatric patients. Options in children are limited and remain experimental but advances in assisted reproduction techniques have focused attention on preserving gonadal tissue for future use [55–59]. Testicular or ovarian tissue could be harvested and stored before sterilising cancer therapy. Following cure, the stored tissue could be autotransplanted, with restoration of natural fertility, or these stored cells could be matured in vitro until they reach a stage sufficiently mature for fertilisation with assisted reproduction. The Royal College of Obstetricians and Gynaecologists and the British Fertility Society have provided reports from the working parties on the storage of ovarian and prepubertal testicular tissue providing standards for best practice in the cryopreservation of gonadal tissue [57]. Cryopreservation of sperm should be offered to young males who will receive gonadotoxic treatments. Semen cryopreservation from young patients (14–17 years of age) is as effective as that from young adults (18–20 years) [58, 59]. Cryopreservation of semen is dependent upon the young patient's ability and willingness to produce a specimen, and consent for storage from a minor will require the patient to be 'Gillick' competent.

The majority of childhood cancer survivors will be fertile, however, counselling patients and families appropriately can be difficult given the varied nature of the treatment. All patients should undergo age-appropriate pubertal staging and further assessment of reproductive function as indicated. In post-pubertal males, a testicular volume of <12 ml, in association with elevated FSH and normal serum testosterone levels, strongly correlates with impaired spermatogenesis. In females, an early follicular phase assay of FSH, oestradiol, and ovarian ultrasound are potential tools to assess ovarian reserve. If there is evidence of ovarian failure, sex steroid replacement therapy is necessary from puberty through to at least the 5th decade for optimal bone mineralisation and cardiovascular protection. In young adult women, physiological sex steroid replacement therapy improves uterine function (blood flow and endometrial thickness) and may potentially enable these women to benefit from assisted reproductive technologies [60, 61].

Cardiac Problems

Both cardiac function and cardiovascular disease can occur as a consequence of treatment for cancer and is associated with increased morbidity and mortality in survivors [62–66]. Early and late cardiac effects are recognised following chemotherapy and radiotherapy including cardiomyopathy, pericarditis, valvular lesions and coronary artery stenosis. Much of these data come from studies in Hodgkin's lymphoma using treatment protocols which have been replaced by new treatment regimens. However, there is substantial evidence that anthracyclines, such as daunorubicin and doxorubicin, cause cardiac damage in a cumulative dose-related fashion [64, 65].The mechanism appears to be focal myocyte death with replacement fibrosis. There is probably no 'safe' anthracycline dose as cardiac dysfunction is reported with relatively low doses and adverse effects increase with time. Younger age at treatment and female gender appear to be independent risk factors [66]. Higher anthracycline doses are also reported to be associated with prolongation of the QT interval [67].

Mediastinal irradiation increases the risk of coronary artery disease and myocardial infarction. Specific risk factors include high dose (>30 Gy), minimal protective cardiac blocking, young age at irradiation and length of follow-up [66]. Patients receiving TBI for bone marrow transplant conditioning must also be considered at risk. Whilst mediastinal radiotherapy appears to induce atheromatous lesions of the proximal coronary arteries (with similar lesions seen in the carotid bulb after cranial irradiation), there is no strong evidence that radiotherapy alters high density lipoprotein lipid levels. Radiation damage has an additive effect to anthracycline cardiotoxicity.

A number of studies of long-term survivors of childhood cancer, at least 5 years after treatment, have found an increase in deaths from cardiovascular disease, with as much as a fivefold excess [68]. In addition to structural changes in the heart and coronary vessels, the entire cardiovascular system appears to be threatened. Survival from childhood cancer is associated with premature evolution of the metabolic syndrome and consequently, an increased risk of cardiovascular mortality and morbidity.

Management of Cardiac Problems

It is recognised that monitoring of cardiovascular risk factors should be a routine part of the long-term care of cancer patients, but the balance between useful and pragmatic assessment of cardiac function is not easy to determine. The literature supports echocardiographic assessment at diagnosis and at regular intervals during treatment. Children who have satisfactory left ventricular function on simple echocardiographic measures and who have received modest anthracycline doses (<250 mg/m^2) may benefit from 3-yearly surveillance. There is no evidence on which to base recommendations for the monitoring of patients who receive higher doses. Early involvement of a cardiologist is essential for patients with an abnormal echocardiogram.

Preliminary investigation of the cardioprotective agent, dexrazoxane, suggested a reduction in the risk of developing short-term subclinical cardiotoxicity; however larger studies are required to substantiate these findings and to explore whether the short-term cardioprotection afforded by dexrazoxane will reduce the incidence of late cardiac complications in survivors of childhood cancer [69–71]. Patients with poor left ventricular function on echocardiogram are generally commenced on ACE inhibitors; however current data do not support this. Although short-term improvements have been demonstrated, studies are uncontrolled, non-blinded, and benefits appear to be transient [71].

Lifestyle changes aimed at reducing these risks, such as weight reduction, regular physical exercise, smoking cessation and healthy eating, should be encouraged. There is no evidence to suggest that restricting employment or limiting activities are beneficial. However, the risks for competitive sporting activity and pregnancy are likely to be considerable and detailed cardiology assessment is recommended for survivors considering becoming pregnant or wishing to take part in competitive sports. Assessment of GH status and lipid profiles is advocated and the therapeutic intervention with GH replacement and lipid-lowering drugs may prevent or delay the development of cardiovascular disease. Lipid-lowering drugs could prevent or delay the onset of cardiovascular disease but there is no evidence available at present to support this.

Renal Morbidity

Renal toxicity after successful treatment of childhood cancer is common and leads to a wide range of manifestations of variable severity, and may be reversible [72, 73]. Causes of nephrotoxicity are multiple, including the disease itself, chemotherapy, radiotherapy, surgery, immunotherapy, and supportive treatment. Assessment of renal toxicity should include both glomerular and renal tubular function. The two most commonly implicated agents are ifosfamide and cis-platinum. Ifosfamide nephrotoxicity predominantly affects the proximal tubule, causing Fanconi syndrome, but may also impair glomerular function. Platinum nephrotoxicity causes glomerular impairment and hypomagnesaemia secondary to tubular damage. Incomplete understanding of the underlying pathogenesis has hindered attempts to develop protective strategies.

Cognitive and Psychosocial Outcomes

Although during the course of cancer treatment children may miss substantial amounts of schooling, a decline in cognitive function is neither a frequent nor inevitable consequence of treatment [74, 75]. However, there is a strong association between cranial irradiation and structural brain abnormalities (disruption of frontal lobe/basal ganglia connections, temporal lobe calcification and cortical atrophy). The functional significance of this is difficult to determine but impairment may be associated with vasculopathy, calcification and EEG abnormalities [75]. Both structural abnormalities and cognitive impairment correlate positively with dose of irradiation and negatively with age at irradiation. Healthcare professionals should be aware that the treatment of childhood cancer may have an impact on neurological function in later life, particularly high dose irradiation and treatment at a young age (SIGN grade D recommendation). Regular review for such deficits should be part of routine follow-up for at-risk patients (SIGN grade D recommendation). Screening at the start of treatment and annually using the Wechsler Intelligence Scale for Children may be helpful. If a problem is suspected children should be referred to a psychologist for further assessment.

Treatment in childhood is likely to impact upon education, psychological and social functioning and thus the impact of overall quality of life. Studies addressing these issues are limited to self-reporting questionnaires. Adverse outcomes with regard to employment and marriage are frequently reported but risk of bias is high. Psychiatric disorders are uncommon but survivors appear to be at increased risk of anxiety, low mood and low self-esteem. Brain tumours and cranial irradiation are frequently reported risk factors for adverse psychological and social outcomes. There are currently no prospective studies using standardised assessment measures which address particular interventions for preventing or managing adverse quality of life outcomes in long-term survivors.

Second Primary Tumours and Tumour Recurrence

One of the most devastating consequences of aggressive cancer therapy is an increased risk of second primary malignancies. Exposure to radiation is associated with a significant risk of developing solid tumours, particularly breast cancer, sarcomas and thyroid cancer. Chemotherapy, particularly the alkylating agents, is known to be associated with development of leukaemia [76–82]. However, our understanding of the long-term risks of second cancers are based on out-dated therapies and there will be an inevitable delay before we can confidently determine the long-term consequences of current therapies. Nevertheless, in the UK, there is a 1 in 25 risk of childhood cancer survivors developing a second primary cancer within 25 years of the primary diagnosis, which is 6 times greater than the general population [76]. It is likely that this relates both to the carcinogenic effects of anti-cancer therapies and a genetic predisposition to cancer development. The excess risk after all childhood cancers (except retinoblastoma) is related to the carcinogenic effects of radiotherapy and the alkylating agents, although there is likely to be some element of genetic predisposition, for example in some families a constitutional mutation of the p53 gene.

Second primary bone cancer affects about 1 in 100 survivors by 20 years from the original diagnosis [77, 78]. Second primary leukaemia is diagnosed in about 1 in 500 childhood cancer survivors in the UK by 6 years from diagnosis, about 8 times the number expected. Increased cumulative exposure to alkylating agents or epipodophyllotoxins increases the risk of subsequent leukaemia [79, 80]. In addition, other topoisomerase II inhibitors, including the anthracyclines, appear leukaemogenic.

Second primary malignancy is the leading cause of death in long-term survivors of Hodgkin's lymphoma. Girls and young women who receive mantle irradiation with greater than 40 Gy have a significantly increased risk of developing breast cancer, with age at time of treatment being the strongest risk factor [81]. The Stanford experience of 885 women followed up for an average of 10 years demonstrated a relative risk of 19.2 (95% CI 10.3–32) for those women treated before age 25 years and a greatly increased relative risk of 136 (95% CI 34–371) for those girls treated before age 15 years. It is important to emphasise that the incidence of breast cancer is very strongly influenced by the dose of radiotherapy. The Stanford group has reported that since the introduction of combined modality therapy over the past 25 years, allowing a reduction in radiotherapy dose and volume, no case of breast cancer has been observed [81, 82].

Developing a Service for the Follow-Up of Long-Term Survivors of Childhood Cancer

With the population of long-term survivors steadily rising and greater awareness of therapy-related morbidity, there is a need to develop a service for the long-term follow-up of survivors of childhood cancer. Recommendations on how to manage some of the late complications of therapy have been discussed above. However, the questions as to who should carry out this surveillance and where, particularly once survivors reach adulthood, remain contentious issues. There is no evidence available to define the optimum setting for the follow-up of long-term survivors. There is good evidence of wide variation in the extent to which survivors of childhood cancer are discharged from hospital follow-up [83]. Many of the adult survivors of childhood cancer are not being followed up and of those under regular surveillance, more than 90% are followed up by the paediatric oncology team in a paediatric oncology unit [84]. Long-term survivors represent a group of young adults who received a variety of different treatment regimens with their attendant side effects profile. Paediatric oncologists, while they may understand the potential side effects, may not be able to offer the appropriate environment or therapy for the young adult. Primary care physicians are inundated with guidelines and policies on many conditions and it would be unrealistic to expect them to have intimate knowledge of cancer therapy and its side effects. The most practical solution is a multidisciplinary team approach between primary and tertiary health professionals.

Awareness of the need to develop a service for the long-term follow-up of cancer survivors is reflected in the recently published guidelines from the UK National Institute for Clinical Excellence (NICE), the Scottish Intercollegiate Guidelines Network (SIGN) and the UK Children's Cancer and Leukaemia Group (CCLG). The approach proposed by NICE, the 'improving outcomes in children and young people with cancer' guidance, involves a long-term follow-up multidisciplinary team (MDT), including a lead clinician with expertise in long-term follow-up (usually an oncologist, but not necessarily paediatric), a specialist nurse, endocrinologist, general practitioner (GP), allied health professionals (e.g. social worker), and a psychologist [85]. Identification of a core team would enable good collaboration between primary and tertiary services and establish early links between the paediatric and adult physicians to ensure the needs of the survivors are met as they become adults. The guidance also recommends that a 'key worker' (probably the specialist nurse) should be identified for each patient to coordinate the care.

While it is recommended that all patients be followed up for life, it is neither necessary nor appropriate that all patients be assessed in a hospital setting. Based on the limited evidence available, the SIGN has developed an evidence-based approach to long-term follow-up [9]. As illustrated in the first section of this chapter, the long-term risks depend upon the underlying malignancy, the site of the tumour, type of treatment and age at time of treatment. Risk-based levels of follow-up were initially described by the CCLG Late Effects Group in 2001, and subsequently incorporated into the SIGN guidelines [6, 9]. Three levels of follow-up, assigned at 5 years off treatment, have been recommended (table 1).

Table 1. Suggested levels of follow-up for long-term survivors of childhood cancer

Level	Treatment	Method of follow-up	Frequency years	Examples of tumours
1	Surgery alone Low risk chemotherapy	Postal or telephone	1–2	Wilms' stage I or II LCH (single-system) Germ cell (surgery only)
2	Chemotherapy Low dose cranial irradiation (≤24 Gy)	Nurse or primary care-led (after appropriated training)	1–2	Majority of patients (e.g. ALL in first remission)
3	Radiotherapy, except low dose cranial irradiation Megatherapy	Medically supervised long-term follow-up clinic	Annual	Brain tumours After bone marrow transplant Any stage 4 patient

'Level 1 follow-up' is recommended for a group of survivors for whom the benefit of clinical follow-up is not clearly established. Annual or even 2-yearly postal or telephone contact may be all that is necessary in order to determine whether there have been adverse health consequences and to enquire about quality of life issues. Level 2 follow-up is for the majority of patients on current protocols, for whom the nature and intensity of follow-up are not easily determined. Nurse- or primary care-led follow-up on an annual basis may suffice although this may miss some individual problems. At the other end of the scale, in level 3 follow-up there are patients who have received radiotherapy (other than low dose cranial irradiation of ≤24 Gy), bone marrow transplantation or megatherapy who will have a significant risk of long-term morbidity. These patients should be seen in a medically supervised long-term follow-up clinic 3–4 times per year until final height is achieved and then annually thereafter. With increasing time from the end of treatment, the risk of developing therapy-related side effects will change and patients can be reassigned an intensity of follow-up at 10 and 15 years off treatment, by which time most survivors will be independent adults. Greater involvement of the general practitioner is integral to this model of care.

The CCLG Late Effects Group [86] recently published a practice statement on therapy-based long-term follow-up, which is designed to inform and guide clinicians responsible for the long-term follow-up of childhood cancer survivors. The practice statement recommends follow-up assessments and investigations based on the treatment that the individual has received and complements the recommendations made by SIGN. In addition, the CCLG have developed a web-based site called 'After Cure' for survivors of childhood cancer [87]. This website provides helpful information on the importance of long-term follow-up, fact sheets on therapy-related late effects, health promotion, and guidance on education, employment and other social issues. This resource should be introduced to patients in the long-term follow-up clinics, with ongoing support from the patient's key worker or nurse specialist.

Implementation of Guidelines

Implementation of guidelines is variable throughout the country and, given the therapy-based approach, long-term follow-up will vary considerably for the different patient groups within each centre. However, there are common strands to long-term follow-up that are applicable to all survivors, including health education and psychosocial support. Currently there is a tendency for hospital dependency for long-term follow-up, often in age-inappropriate settings. This culture is felt to be potentially detrimental to patients in terms of discouraging independence, rehabilitation and empowerment, in addition to inappropriate use of overstretched resources. Stratification of patients according to risk of late morbidity will maximise the use of resources and provide age-appropriate care as locally as possible. With increasing time from completion of treatment, it is hoped that the majority of adult survivors will be independent and take responsibility for their own health, with healthcare support provided by primary care.

Transitioning Paediatric Patients into the Adult Services

Survivors have traditionally been followed up in paediatric clinics long into adulthood. This is not only an age-inappropriate environment for these patients, but also an unsustainable situation for paediatric oncologists, as the population of long-term survivors increases and ages. At present, input from adult physicians for long-term survivors is generally provided in endocrine or neurology clinics; however, for many patients other chronic problems may be missed and left untreated. It is anticipated that with the development of the long-term follow-up MDT and greater collaboration between paediatricians, adult physicians and primary care this will change. Realistically, most children will continue to be followed up in the paediatric hospital setting either in nurse-led or paediatric oncology-led clinics until they have been off treatment for 10 years, or reach adulthood. Between 5 and 10 years after treatment patients and parents should be educated about any potential cancer- or therapy-related problems the child may experience in the future. Patients/parents should be provided with a treatment summary card and advised of the relevant supporting websites (e.g., www.aftercure.co.uk). A patient treatment summary should also be sent to the patient's family doctor to optimise communication and ensure the family doctor is fully equipped to play his/her role in the multidisciplinary long-term follow-up of survivors.

Assigning a Level of Follow-Up for Patients of Transition Age (16–18 Years)
One of the major difficulties for a paediatric oncologist responsible for the long-term follow-up of patients has been how to transition young adults from paediatric services into the appropriate adult setting. Young adult survivors (aged 16–18 years) can be reassigned a level of follow-up to enable them to be transitioned into the age-appropriate services.

For patients assigned level 1 follow-up, the late-effects nurse will continue to liaise with them either by telephone or postal questionnaire. It will be essential to ensure that GPs are kept up to date with outcomes from postal questionnaires and offer survivors the opportunity for review, either by their GP, or the hospital-based late-effects clinic.

For patients assigned level 2, it is recommended that patients be followed up by their GP or attend nurse-led late-effects clinic. Although the risks of developing late sequelae are small for these patients, a number of them will require on-going surveillance by the GP or specialist late-effects nurse. With time, it is recommended that this hospital clinic be in an adult setting run by a specialist late-effects nurse.

Many patients will have received treatment that is associated with a significant risk of developing late side effects, which may or may not be evident by the time a patient is 16–18 years of age and will require ongoing hospital-based follow-up: level 3. Children who develop treatment-related side effects, particularly endocrine or neurological problems, will be seen by an endocrinologist or neurologist as part of a paediatric joint late-effects clinic. Upon reaching adulthood, those patients who have already developed therapy-related complications, at least part of their care, can be transferred to the appropriate adult specialists. However, for many patients complications may not yet be evident or there is a risk of complications other than endocrine or neurological problems, which will not generally be screened for in a specialist adult clinic. Hence, there is a need for multidisciplinary long-term follow-up of all level 3 patients, co-ordinated by a clinician with an understanding of the late effects of childhood cancer treatment. Management of adult survivors should take place in an adult environment with on-going support from the paediatric oncologist and late-effects nurse specialist.

A small number of survivors with a limited spectrum of complications may be followed up only by the appropriate adult specialist, obviating the need for another hospital visit to attend a late-effects clinic. The health status of these patients will of course continue to be monitored by postal questionnaires as we believe that it is important for paediatric oncologists to have an understanding of the long-term health of patients treated for childhood cancer.

Role of the General Practitioner

The primary care team is likely to play an increasing role in the long-term follow-up of survivors of childhood cancer. Primary care services may already be stretched but GPs are used to meet targets and ensure guidelines are implemented. Good communication between hospital services and primary care will be essential. Early involvement of GPs in the long-term follow-up MDT will establish collaborations between the 2 teams and enable GPs to become familiar with the surveillance programme. The feasibility of GPs taking on the additional responsibility or late effects of childhood cancer surveillance has yet to be evaluated in the UK. However, data to support the greater involvement of GPs in the follow-up of adult survivors has recently been published by a Dutch group. Blaauwbroek et al. [88] demonstrated that shared care by paediatric oncologists and family doctors is feasible for the long-term follow-up of survivors of childhood cancer. Over a 3-year period, 123 or 133 (92%) randomly selected adults (from 210 five-year survivors of childhood cancer, excluding CNS tumours and single-site Langerhans cell histiocytosis) were successfully followed up annually by paediatric oncologist, alternating with their family doctors. Assessment of late effects was based upon the UKCCLG Late Effects Group guidelines and late complications graded according to the Common Terminology for Adverse Events. Furthermore, they showed that shared care is compatible with the collection of data required for cancer registration and more than 80% of family doctors and survivors were satisfied with the model of care [88].

Developing the Role of the Late-Effects Nurse Specialist

The late-effects nurse specialist (LENS) can play an integral role in the multidisciplinary team follow-up of long-term survivors of childhood cancer. Their initial role would be to assist with a retrospective phase of the project and to develop a patient database. The LENS can identify and contact patients lost to follow-up and, henceforth, ensure that the patient receives appropriate future follow-up. The nurse specialist would co-ordinate and support the completion of health status and well being questionnaires, by post, telephone or in hospital clinics.

The LENS should play an important role in preparing level 1 patients for the step towards independence. However, educating the patient to take responsibility for ongoing surveillance is unlikely to be sufficient in many cases. Completion of a health status questionnaire (with the assistance of the LENS) may provide an opportunity to prompt patients to attend their GPs for review. The LENS can play a key role in educating patients/parents during the transition period from paediatric-based to adult-based services and will ensure that patients are not lost to follow-up.

Conclusions

Survivors of childhood cancer are at significant risk of developing late complications following the successful treatment of their cancer during childhood. Increasing awareness of the late complications of cancer therapy dictates vigilant long-term follow-up of these patients with early intervention, institution of treatment where appropriate, and appropriate counselling. The evidence base to guide the establishment of a structure for long-term clinical follow-up is incomplete and current best practice is that all survivors should be followed up for life. In the UK, strategies are currently being developed to define a comprehensive programme for follow-up together with centralising of data to evaluate the late effects of childhood cancer therapy in the expectation that future treatment protocols may be modified where possible. The British Childhood Cancer Survivor Study will investigate the risks of particular adverse health outcomes occurring amongst survivors and their offspring and relate outcomes to treatment modalities. In this review we present the evidence available on the late complications following chemotherapy and radiotherapy treatment and make recommendations for the long-term follow-up of survivors of childhood cancer.

References

1 Campbell J, Wallace WH, Bhatti LA, Stockton DL, Brewster DH: Cancer in Scotland: trends in incidence, mortality and survival 1975–1999. Edinburgh, Information and Statistics Division. www.isdscotland.org/cancer_information.

2 Robison LL, Mertens AC, Boice JD, et al: Study design and cohort characteristics of the Childhood Cancer Survivor Study: a multi-institutional collaborative project. Med Pediatr Oncol 2002;38: 229–239.

3 Mertens AC, Yasui Y, Neglia JP, et al: Late mortality experience in five-year survivors of childhood and adolescent cancer: the Childhood Cancer Survivor Study. J Clin Oncol 2001;19:3163–3172.

4 Parkes SE, Jenkinson HC, Griffiths A, Kinch D, Mann JR: Is postal follow-up of childhood cancer survivors worthwhile? Pediatr Blood Cancer 2008; 50:80–84.

5 Oeffinger KC, Mertens AC, Sklar CA, et al: Childhood Cancer Survivor Study. Chronic health conditions in adult survivors of childhood cancer. N Engl J Med 2006;355:1572–1582.

6 Wallace WHB, Blacklay A, Eiser C, et al: Developing strategies for long term follow up of survivors of childhood cancer. BMJ 2001;323:271–274.

7 Blaauwbroek R, Groenier KH, Kamps WA, Meyboom-de Jong B, Postma A: Late effects in adult survivors of childhood cancer: the need for lifelong follow-up. Ann Oncol 2007;18:1898–1902.

8 Landier W, Wallace WH, Hudson MM: Long-term follow-up of childhood cancer survivors: education, surveillance, and screening. Pediatr Blood Cancer 2006;46:149–158.

9 Scottish Intercollegiate Guidelines Network (SIGN): Long term follow up of survivors of childhood cancer. Guideline No. 76 (SIGN 2004) www.sign.ac.uk.

10 SIGN. SIGN 50 – A guideline developers handbook. Scottish Intercollegiate Guidelines Network, 2002. www.sign.ac.uk/guidelines/fulltext/ 50/index.html.

11 Oberfield SE, Sklar CA: Endocrine sequelae in survivors of childhood cancer. Adolesc Med 2002; 13:161–169.

12 Clayton PE, Shalet SM, Morris-Jones PH, Price DA: Growth in children treated for acute lymphoblastic leukaemia. Lancet 1988;i:460–462.

13 Crowne EC, Moore C, Wallace WHB, et al. A novel variant of growth hormone insufficiency following low dose cranial irradiation. Clin Endocrinol (Oxf) 1992;36:59–68.

14 Ogilvy-Stuart AL, Clark DJ, Wallace WH, et al: Endocrine deficit after fractionated total body irradiation. Arch Dis Child 1992;67:1107–1110.
15 Littley MD, Shalet SM, Beardwell CG, et al: Hypopituitarism following external radiotherapy for pituitary tumours in adults. Q J Med 1989; 70:145–160.
16 Shalet SM, Gibson B, Swindell R, et al: Effect of spinal irradiation on growth. Arch Dis Child 1987; 62:461–464.
17 Holm K, Nysom K, Rasmussen MH, Hertz H, Jacobsen N, Skakkebaek NE, Krabbe S, Müller J: Growth, growth hormone and final height after BMT. Possible recovery of irradiation-induced growth hormone insufficiency. Bone Marrow Transplant 1996;18:163–170.
18 Darzy KH, Shalet SM: Radiation-induced growth hormone deficiency. Horm Res 2003;59(suppl 1):1–11.
19 Livesey EA, Hindmarsh PC, Brook CG, Whitton AC, Bloom HJ, Tobias JS, Godlee JN, Britton J: Endocrine disorders following treatment of childhood brain tumors. Br J Cancer 1990;61:622–625.
20 Brennan BM, Mughal Z, Roberts SA, et al: Bone mineral density in childhood survivors of acute lymphoblastic leukemia treated without cranial irradiation. J Clin Endocrinol Metab 2005;90: 689–694.
21 Crofton PM, Ahmed SF, Wade JC, et al: Effects of intensive chemotherapy on bone and collagen turnover and the growth hormone axis in children with acute lymphoblastic leukaemia. J Clin Endocrinol Metab 1998;83:3121–3129.
22 Ahmed SF, Wallace WHB, Kelnar CJH: An anthropometric study of children during intensive chemotherapy for acute lymphoblastic leukaemia. Horm Res 1997;48:178–183.
23 Ahmed SF, Wallace WHB, Crofton PM, et al: Short term changes in lower leg length in children treated for acute lymphoblastic leukaemia. J Pediatr Endocrinol Metabol 1999;12:75–80.
24 Crofton PM, Ahmed SF, Wade JC, et al: Effects of a third intensification block of chemotherapy on bone and collagen turnover, insulin-like growth factors I, its binding proteins and short term growth in children with acute lymphoblastic leukaemia. Eur J Cancer 1999;35:960–967.
25 Crofton PM, Ahmed SF, Wade JC, et al: Bone turnover and growth during and after continuing therapy in children with acute lymphoblastic leukaemia. Pediatr Res 2000;48:490–496.
26 Swerdlow AJ, Reddingius RE, Higgins CD, et al: Growth hormone treatment of children with brain tumours and risk of tumour recurrence. J Clin Endocrinol Metab 2000;85:4444–4449.
27 Reilly JJ, Ventham JC, Newell J, et al: Risk factors for excessive weight gain in children treated for acute lymphoblastic leukaemia. Int J Obes Relat Metab Disord 2000;24:1537–1541.
28 Scottish Intercollegiate Guidelines Network (SIGN): Management of Obesity in Children and Young People. Edinburgh, SIGN, 2003, No. 69. www.sign.ac.uk.
29 Ron E, Modan B, Preston D, et al: Thyroid neoplasia following low-dose radiation on the pituitary and thyroid glands. Radiat Res 1989;120: 516–531.
30 Livesey EA, Brook CG: Thyroid dysfunction after radiotherapy and chemotherapy of childhood brain tumours. Arch Dis Child 1989;64:593–595.
31 Sklar CA, Mertens AC, Walter A, et al: Changes in body mass index and prevalence of overweight in survivors of childhood acute lymphoblastic leukemia: role of cranial irradiation. Med Pediatr Oncol 2000;35:91–95.
32 Inskip PD: Thyroid cancer after radiotherapy for childhood cancer. Med Pediatr Oncol 2001;36: 568–573.
33 Pottern LM, Kaplan MM, Larsen PR, et al: Thyroid nodularity after childhood irradiation for lymphoid hyperplasia: a comparison of questionnaire and clinical findings. J Clin Epidemiol 1990; 43:449–460.
34 Constine LS, Woolf PD, Cann D, et al: Hypothalamic-pituitary dysfunction after radiation for brain tumors. N Engl J Med 1993;328:87–94.
35 Ogilvy-Stuart AL, Clayton PE, Shalet SM. Cranial irradiation and early puberty. J Clin Endocrinol Metab 1994;78:1282–6.
36 Leiper AD, Stanhope R, Preece MA, Grant DB, Chessells JM: Precocious or early puberty and growth failure in girls treated for acute lymphoblastic leukaemia. Horm Res 1988;30:72–76.
37 Bath LE, Anderson RA, Critchley HO, et al: Hypothalamic-pituitary-ovarian dysfunction after prepubertal chemotherapy and cranial irradiation for acute leukaemia. Hum Reprod 2001;16: 1838–1844.
38 Mackie EJ, Radford M, Shalet SM: Gonadal function following chemotherapy for childhood Hodgkin's disease. Med Pediatr Oncol 1996;27: 74–78.
39 Speiser B, Rubin P, Casarett G: Azoospermia following lower truncal irradiation in Hodgkin's disease. Cancer 1973;32:692–696.

40 Clifton DK, Bremner WJ: The effect of testicular X-irradiation on spermatogenesis in man. A comparison with the mouse. J Androl 1983;6:387–392.
41 Rowley MJ, Leach DR, Warner GA, Heller CG: Effects of graded ionising radiation on the human testis. Radiat Res 1974;59:665–678.
42 Shalet SM, Horner A, Ahmed SR, et al: Leydig cell function after testicular irradiation for lymphoblastic leukaemia. Horm Res 1985;30:53–61.
43 Shalet SM, Tsatsoulis A, Whitehead E, Read G: Vulnerability of the human Leydig cell to radiation damage is dependent upon age. J Endocrinol 1989;120:161–165.
44 Hawkins MM, Draper GJ, Smith RA: Cancer among 1348 survivors of childhood cancer. Int J Cancer 1989;43:975–978.
45 Li FP, Fine W, Jaffe N, et al: Offspring of patients treated for cancer in childhood. J Natl Cancer Inst 1979;62:1193–1197.
46 Sutcliffe AG, Taylor B, Saunders K, Thornton S, Lieberman BA: Outcome in the second year of life after in-vitro fertilisation by intracytoplasmic sperm injection: a UK case-control study. Lancet 2001;357:2080–2084.
47 Thomson AB, Irvine DS, Campbell AJ, Anderson RA, Kelnar CJH, Wallace WHB: Semen quality and spermatozoal DNA integrity in survivors of childhood cancer: a case-control study. Lancet 2002;360:361–367.
48 Wallace WHB, Thomson AB, Kelsey T: The radiosensitivity of the human oocyte. Hum Reprod 2003;323:271–274.
49 Wallace WH, Thomson AB, Saran F, Kelsey TW: Predicting age of ovarian failure after radiation to a field that includes the ovaries. Int J Radiat Oncol Biol Phys 2005;62:738–744.
50 Critchley HO, Wallace WH: Impact of cancer treatment on uterine function. J Natl Cancer Inst Monogr 2005;34:64–68.
51 Green DM, Whitton JA, Stovall M, et al: Pregnancy outcome of female survivors of childhood cancer: a report from the Childhood Cancer Survivor Study. Am J Obst Gynecol 2002;1887:1070–1080.
52 Critchley HO, Wallace WB, Shalet SM, Mamtora H, Higginson J, Anderson DC: Abdominal irradiation in childhood: potential for pregnancy. Br J Gynaecol 1992;99:392–394.
53 Edgar AB, Wallace WH: Pregnancy in women who had cancer in childhood. Eur J Cancer 2007; 43:1890–1894.
54 Crofton PM, Thomson AB, Evans AE, et al: Is inhibin B a potential marker of gonadotoxicity in prepubertal children treated for cancer. Clin Endocrinol (Oxf) 2003;58:296–301.
55 Shaw JM, Bowles J, Koopman P, et al: Fresh and cryopreserved ovarian tissue samples from donors with lymphoma transmit the cancer to the graft recipients. Hum Reprod 1996;11:1668–1673.
56 Grundy R, Larcher V, Gosden RG, et al: Personal practice: fertility preservation for children treated for cancer (2): ethics of consent for gamete storage and experimentation. Arch Dis Child 2001;84: 360–362.
57 Royal College of Obstetricians and Gynaecologists: Storage of Ovarian and Prepubertal Testicular Tissue: Report of a Working Party. London, Royal College of Obstetricians and Gynaecologists, 2000.
58 Kliesch S, Behre HM, Jurgens H, Nieschlag E: Cryopreservation of semen from adolescent patients with malignancies. Med Pediatr Oncol 1996;26:20–27.
59 Lass A, Akagbosu F, Abusheikha N, et al: A programme of semen cryopreservation for patients with malignant disease in a tertiary infertility centre: lessons from 8 years' experience. Hum Reprod 1998;13:3256–3261.
60 Critchley HO, Buckley CH, Anderson DC: Experience with a 'physiological' steroid replacement regimen for the establishment of a receptive endometrium in women with premature ovarian failure. Br J Obstet Gynaecol 1990;97:804–810.
61 Bath LE, Critchley HO, Chambers SE, et al: Ovarian and uterine characteristics after total body irradiation in childhood: response to sex steroid replacement. Br J Obstet Gynaecol 1999;106: 1265–1272.
62 Bu'Lock FA, Mott MG, Oakhill A, Martin RP: Left ventricular diastolic function after anthracycline chemotherapy in childhood: relation with systolic function, symptoms, and pathophysiology. Br Heart J 1995;73:340–350.
63 Lipshultz SE, Lipsitz SR, Mone SM, et al: Female sex and drug dose as risk factors for late cardiotoxic effects of doxorubicin therapy for childhood cancer. N Engl J Med 1995;332:1738–1743.
64 Sorensen K, Levitt G, Bull C, et al: Anthracycline dose in childhood acute lymphoblastic leukaemia: issues of early survival versus late cardiotoxicity. J Clin Oncol 1997;15:61–68.
65 Sorensen K, Levitt GA, Bull C, et al: Late anthracycline toxicity after childhood cancer: a prospective longitudinal study. Cancer 2003;97: 1991–1998.

66 Hancock SL, Tucker MA, Hope RT: Factors affecting late mortality from heart disease after treatment for Hodgkin's disease. JAMA 1993;270: 1949–1955.

67 Schwartz CL, Hobbie WL, Truesdaell S, et al: Corrected QT interval prolongation in anthracycline-treated survivors of childhood cancer. J Clin Oncol 1993;11:1906–1910.

68 Talvensaari KK, Lanning M, Tapanainen P, Knip M: Long-term survivors of childhood cancer have an increased risk of manifesting the metabolic syndrome. J Clin Endocrinol Metab 1996;81: 3051–3055.

69 Wexler LH, Andrich MP, Venzon D, et al: Randomised trial of the cardioprotective agent ICRF 187 in paediatric sarcoma patients treated with doxorubicin. J Clin Oncol 1996;14:362–372.

70 Lipshultz SE, Rifai N, Dalton VM, et al: The effect of dexrazoxane on myocardial injury in doxorubicin-treated children with acute lymphoblastic leukemia. N Engl J Med 2004;351:145–153.

71 Bryant J, Picot J, Levitt G, Sullivan I, Baxter L, Clegg A: Cardioprotection against the toxic effects of anthracyclines given to children with cancer: a systematic review. Health Technol Assess 2007;11:iii, ix–x, 1–84.

72 Skinner R, Cotterill SJ, Stevens MC: Risk factors for nephrotoxicity after ifosfamide treatment in children: a UKCCSG Late Effects Group study. United Kingdom Children's Cancer Study Group. Br J Cancer 2000;82:1636–1645.

73 Kilbridge BR, Morris-Jones PH, Addison GM: Prevention of cisplatin-induced hypomagnesemia. Pediatr Hematol Oncol 1988;5:1–6.

74 Eiser C, Hill JJ, Vance YH: Examining the psychological consequences of surviving childhood cancer: systematic review as a research method in pediatric psychology. J Pediatr Psychol 2000;25: 449–460.

75 Mulhern RK, Reddick WE, Palmer SL, et al: Neurocognitive deficits in medulloblastoma survivors and white matter loss. Ann Neurol 1999;46:834–841.

76 Hawkins MM, Draper GJ, Kingston JE: Incidence of second primary tumours among childhood cancer survivors. Br J Cancer 1987;56:339–347.

77 Hawkins MM, Kinnier Wilson LM, Burton HS, et al: Radiotherapy, alkylating agents and the risk of bone cancer after childhood cancer. J Natl Cancer Inst 1996;88:270–278.

78 Tucker MA, D'Agio GJ, Boice JD, et al: Bone sarcomas linked to radiotherapy and chemotherapy in children. N Engl J Med 1987;317:588–593.

79 Tucker MA, Meadows AT, Boice JD, et al: Leukaemia after therapy with alkylating agents for childhood cancer. J Natl Cancer Inst 1987;78:459–464.

80 Hawkins MM, Kinnier Wilson LM, Stovall MA, et al: Epidophyllotoxins, alkylating agents, and radiation and risk of secondary leukaemia after childhood cancer. BMJ 1992;304:951–958.

81 Hancock SL, Tucker MA, Hoppe RT: Breast cancer after treatment of Hodgkin's disease. J Natl Cancer Inst 1993;85:25–31.

82 Donaldson SS, Hancock SL, Hoppe RT: Hodgkin's disease – finding the balance between cure and late effects. Cancer J Sci Am 1999;5:325–333.

83 Taylor A, Hawkins M, Blacklay A, et al: Long term follow up of survivors of childhood cancer in the UK. Paediatr Blood Cancer 2004;42:161–168.

84 Oeffinger KC, Eshelman DA, Tomlinson GE, Buchanan GR: Programs for adult survivors of childhood cancer. J Clin Oncol 1998;16:292–297.

85 NICE Guidance on Cancer Services: Improving Outcomes in Children and Young People with Cancer. London, National Collaborating Centre for Cancer 2005. www.nice.org.uk.

86 Kissen GDN, Wallace WHB (eds): United Kingdom Children's Cancer Study Group (now known as Children's Cancer and Leukaemia Group (CCLG)), Late Effects Group: Therapy-Based Long-Term Follow-Up Practice Statement, ed 2. Leicester, CCLG, 2005.

87 Children's Cancer and Leukaemia Group (CCLG). www.aftercure.org.

88 Blaauwbroek R, Tuinier W, Meyboom-de Jong B, et al: Shared care by paediatric oncologists and family doctors for long-term follow-up of adult childhood cancer survivors: a pilot study Lancet Oncol 2008:9:232–238.

Dr. Angela B. Edgar
Department of Haematology/Oncology, Royal Hospital for Sick Children
17 Millerfield Place
Edinburgh EH9 1LW (UK)
Tel. +44 131 536 0420, Fax +44 131 536 0430, E-Mail angela.edgar@luht.scot.nhs.uk

Subject Index